Intermittent Fasting 16/8

The Ultimate Step-By-Step Guide To 8-Hour Diet, Which Makes You Live Healthy, Lose Weight, Burn Fat and Age Slowly with Autophagy and Metabolism, Including Recipes

By Asuka Young

Table of Contents

Introduction

Intermittent Fasting (IF) is known to be the dietary eating patterns, which include a prolonged period of not eating or severely restricting calories. There are many different intermittent fasting subgroups, each with individual differences in the length of the fast; some for hours, some for day(s). This has become a prevalent subject within the scientific community due to all the potential benefits that are being found in terms of fitness and safety.

There are no excuses for not moving. People often think they have no other option than to keep gaining weight, but maintaining the ideal weight is essential for health. Even losing weight in the right way is equally important.

Being overweight or clinically obese means having a high caloric intake and low energy expenditure. To lose weight, it is important to reduce calorie intake both with the diet and by practicing regular physical activity because the diet is always more effective when combined with movement. In any case, combining physical activity makes the diet more and more effective.

Many people work out to lose weight, but they do it the wrong way because they think that intense cardio exercise or prolonged sessions allow them to lose weight faster and keep the extra pounds away. This method actually turns out to be ineffective. In order not to lose the benefits of training, it is important to watch your diet more closely.

A widespread habit among those who want to lose weight is to practice fasting. If on one hand, it can be an advantage, on the other it is risky for health. The recommended duration of fasting aerobic activity is about 40 minutes; beyond this duration, it is possible to resort to the consumption of stock proteins, with consequent muscle catabolism, that is, destruction of muscle mass.

It is natural to reduce the amount of food taken to decrease calorie intake. However, adopting a regulated food intake, such as diets based only on the consumption of fruit and vegetables and eliminating certain foods altogether has been proven more effective than other methods of weight loss. In this cookbook, we present recipes, which can make you lose weight pretty fast and more effectively without any form of side effect.

Physical activity and nutrition are two main complementary elements. To lose weight intelligently, you need to combine the right amount of physical activity with a correct diet.

Chapter 1:

What Is Intermittent Fasting (IF)?

Intermittent fasting (IF) is the pattern of eating, which cycles between fasting and eating periods.It does not dictate what foods to consume, but rather when to eat. It's not a diet in a conventional manner, but more accurately described as a method of eating in this way.

Common methods of intermittent fasting involve 16-hour daily fasts or 24-hour fasting, twice a week. Fasting was a practice throughout all of human evolution. Ancient hunter-gatherers didn't have all-year-round supermarkets, refrigerators, or milk. They were sometimes unable to find anything to cook.

As a consequence, humans evolved to be able to function for extended periods without food. It is more natural to fast regularly than always eating 3–4 (or more) meals a day. Fasting is also often carried out for religious or spiritual purposes, in Islam, Christianity, Judaism, and Buddhism, among others.

Intermittent Fasting Methods

There are several ways to do intermittent fasting— all of which involve splitting the day or week into periods of eating and fasting.During the periods of fasting, you either eat very little or nothing.

Those methods are the most popular:

The 16/8 method: It is often known as the Leangains protocol, which involves skipping breakfast and restricting the average meal time to 8 hours, such as 1–9 pm. Then you'll fast in between for 16 hours.

Eat-Stop-Eat: It includes a 24-hour fast, once or twice a week, e.g., by not eating dinner one day and fasting till the dinner of the next day.

The 5:2 diet: With these approaches, on two non-consecutive days of the week, you consume just 500–600 calories but normally eat the other five days. By lowering the intake of calories, all of these strategies will cause weight loss as long as you don't compensate by eating any more during the feeding time. The 16/8 approach is considered by many to be the most straightforward, most effective, and easy to adhere to. It is the most common one, too.

How It Affects Your Cells and Hormones

When you abstain from eating, many things happen in your body both on the cellular and molecular level. As an example, the body adjusts the hormonal levels to make it more accessible to accumulated body fat. Often, the cells start critical mechanisms of restoring and altering gene expression.

Here are some changes happening in your body when you're fasting:

Human Growth Hormone (HGH): Growth hormone levels surge, rising as much as 5-fold. This has advantages in terms of fat loss and muscle gain, to name a few.

Insulin: Insulin sensitivity increases and insulin levels drop dramatically. Higher insulin levels improve the sensitivity of retained body fat.

Cellular repair: The cells start cellular reparation processes when they fast. This involves autophagy, in which cells digest and remove old and damaged proteins that develop within cells.

Gene expression: There are variations in gene expression associated with survival and disease prevention. Such changes in hormone levels, cell function, and gene expression are responsible for intermittent fasting's health benefits.

A Very Powerful Weight Loss Tool

Weight loss is the most prominent reason people seek intermittent fasting. IF can lead to an automatic reduction in calorie intake by making you eat fewer meals. Intermittent fasting adjusts the rates of the hormones that promote weight loss. It increases the production of the fat-burning hormone norepinephrine (noradrenaline) in addition to reducing insulin and raising growth hormone levels.

Because of these hormone changes, the metabolic rate can be raised by 3.6–14 percent in the short term. Intermittent fasting promotes weight loss by shifting all sides of the calorie equation and making you eat less and burn more calories. Studies have shown intermittent fasting can be a powerful tool for weight loss.

A 2014 research study found that this style of eating would cause weight loss of 3–8 percent over 3–24 weeks, which is a significant amount relative to most studies of weight loss. Participants have lost 4–7 percent of their waist circumference, suggesting a significant loss of unhealthy belly fat that develops around the organs and causes disease, according to the same report.

The study showed that intermittent fasting produces less loss of muscle than the more standard method of daily restriction of calories.

Keep in mind, however, that the main reason for their popularity is that intermittent fasting makes you eat fewer overall calories. If you binge during eating periods and eat massive amounts, you may not lose any weight at all.

Health Benefits

There have been many reports on intermittent fasting in animals as well as in humans. Such findings have shown that it can have significant benefits on your body and brain for weight control and wellbeing. It can even make you go on living longer.

Here are the most significant health effects of intermittent fasting:

Weight loss: As described above, intermittent fasting will help you lose weight and fat on your butt, without deliberately restricting calories.

Insulin resistance: IF can reduce insulin resistance, lower blood sugar by 3–6 percent, and fast insulin levels by 20–31 percent, which should protect against type 2 diabetes.

Inflammation: Several studies show decreases in inflammatory levels, which are a vital driver of many chronic diseases.

Heart health: Intermittent fasting will decrease "poor" LDL cholesterol, triglycerides in the blood, inflammatory markers, blood sugar, and tolerance to insulin— all risk factors for heart disease.

Cancer: Studies show that intermittent fasting also prevents cancer.

Brain health: Intermittent fasting raises the BDNF brain hormone and may help new nerve cells to grow. It could also guard against the condition of Alzheimer's.

Anti-aging: Intermittent fasting can prolong the rat lifespan. Research has shown that fasted rats live longer than 36–83 percent of non-fasted rats.

Remember, research is still in its early stages. Many of the experiments have been small, short-term, or carried out in livestock. For higher quality human studies, several questions are yet to be resolved.

Chapter 2:

16/8 Intermittent Fasting

For thousands of years, fasts have been practiced and are a tradition across many diverse religions and cultures around the world.

Today, modern fasting variations put a new spin on the old practice.

16/8: One of the most popular styles of fasting is intermittent fasting. Proponents claim that weight loss and overall health improvements are an easy, convenient and sustainable way to do so.

This chapter reviews intermittent fasting on 16/8, how it works, and if it's right for you.

What Is 16/8 Intermittent Fasting?

16/8 Intermittent fasting means restricting the consumption of food and calorie-containing drinks to a fixed eight-hour window per day and abstaining from the remainder of the 16 hours from eating.

Depending on your personal choice, this process can be repeated as often as you like — from just once or twice a week to every day.

In recent years, 16/8 intermittent fasting has skyrocketed in popularity, especially among those looking to lose weight and burn fat.

While other diets also set strict rules and regulations, intermittent 16/8 fasting is easy to follow and can provide minimal effort to produce real results.

It is generally regarded as less rigid and more flexible than many other diet plans, and can easily fit into almost any lifestyle.

In addition to enhancing weight loss, it is also believed that 16/8 intermittent fasting will improve blood sugar, boost brain function and improve longevity.

How to Get Started

16/8 Simple, safe and sustainable intermittent fasts.

To get started, first pick an eight-hour window and limit your food intake to that period.

Most people prefer to eat between midday and 8 p.m., as this means that you only need to run overnight and skip breakfast, but you can still eat a balanced lunch and dinner and a few snacks all day long.

Many tend to eat at 9 a.m. Then 5 p.m., leaving plenty of time for a healthy breakfast at 9 a.m., a regular lunch at midday and a light early dinner or snack at 4 p.m.

Before starting your fast, you should experiment with and pick the time frame that best fits your schedule.

Everything you eat, it's recommended that you eat multiple small meals and snacks evenly spaced all day long to help stabilize blood sugar levels and keep appetite under control.

Additionally, it is essential to stick to nutritious whole foods and beverages during your eating periods to maximize diet potential health benefits.

Filling in foods that are rich in nutrients can help you complete your diet and enable you to reap the rewards this diet has to offer.

Try balancing each meal with a tasty variety of whole, healthy foods, like:

Fruits, e.g. apples, bananas, berries, oranges, peaches, pears, etc.

Veggies, e.g. broccoli, cauliflower, cucumbers, leafy greens, tomatoes, etc.

Whole grains, e.g. quinoa, rice, oats, barley, buckwheat, etc.

Healthy fats, e.g. Olive oil

Sources of proteins, e.g. meat, poultry, fish, legumes, eggs, nuts, seeds, etc.

Drinking calorie-free drinks, such as water and unsweetened tea and coffee, can also help control your appetite while keeping you hydrated even while fasting.

Also, binging or overdoing it on junk food can negate the positive effects of 16/8 intermittent fasting and can end up doing more harm to your health than good.

Benefits of 16/8 Intermittent Fasting

16/8 Intermittent fasting is an everyday diet because it is easy to follow, versatile and long-term sustainable.

It's also easy, as it can cut down on how much time and money you need to spend each week on cooking and preparing food.

16/8 intermittent fasting has been linked to a long list of benefits in terms of health, including:

Increased weight loss: Not only does it help to cut calories for the day by restricting the intake to a few hours a day, but also it could boost metabolism and weight loss, studies have revealed.

Improved blood sugar: Intermittent fasting has been shown to reduce the risk of diabetes by up to 31 percent and lower blood sugar by 3–6 percent.

Enhanced longevity: Although evidence in humans is limited, some animal studies have found that longevity may be extended by intermittent fasting.

Is 16/8 Intermittent Fasting Right for Me?

16/8 Intermittent fasting in combination with a nutritious diet and a healthy lifestyle can be a sustainable, safe and easy way to improve your health.

It should not, however, be seen as a replacement for a healthy, well-rounded diet rich in whole foods. Not to mention, even if intermittent fasting isn't working for you, you can still be healthy.

Although intermittent fasting of 16/8 is generally considered safe for most healthy adults, you should speak with your doctor before trying it, especially if you have any underlying health conditions.

This is critical if you take any medications or have asthma, low blood pressure or a history of eating disorders.

IF is also not recommended for women who try to conceive, or get pregnant or breastfeeding women.

Always consult your doctor if you have any concerns or experience any adverse side effects while fasting.

Summary

16/8 Intermittent fasting involves eating only for 8 hours and fasting for the remaining 16 hours.

It can facilitate weight loss and improve blood sugar, brain function and lifespan.

During your mealtime, eat a healthy diet and drink calorie-free drinks such as water or unsweetened teas and coffee.

Before embarking on intermittent fasting, it is best to speak with your doctor, particularly if you have any underlying health problems.

Chapter 3:

Is 16:8 Fasting Good For Weight Loss?

Different studies have found that there is virtually no difference between people who observed intermittent fasting regularly and those who cut back their overall calorie intake.

A developing body of research shows that a better strategy is to optimize the nutritional rate of what has been eaten (veggies, fruit, lean protein, whole grains, and healthy fats), as opposed to fasting or calorie counting. Science also shows that any potential benefit from fasting is easily lost during the cycle's feeding phase, where appetite-suppressing hormones switch gears and make you feel even hungrier than you did at baseline.

But some dietitians may benefit from day-to-day fasting if they have difficulty adhering to prescribed meal plans; a 2018 pilot study published in the Journal of Nutrition and Safe Eating shows that a 16:8 fasting program may help obese dietitians lose weight by counting every single calorie they consume. This fasting approach might also help those struggling with other weight-related issues— high blood pressure, in particular. A recent academic analysis published in the New England Journal of Medicine indicates that a 16:8 fasting strategy may help the body to naturally improve the control of blood sugar, as well as reduce overall blood pressure over the long term.

Is fasting 16 hours a day healthy?

Intermittent fasting forms such as the 16:8 diet rely on the concept that fasting reduces oxidative stress on the body, which can reduce inflammation and chronic disease risk.

It's also theorized that, according to a recent study published in Cell Metabolism, fasting gives the important organs, digestive and absorptive hormones, and metabolic functions a "break". Since our bodies secrete insulin to help our cells absorb sugar, over time, fasting is associated with reducing our susceptibility to insulin resistance. (In the end, high levels of insulin put us at risk for a whole host of diseases.) However, research also linked fasting with increases in LDL cholesterol (the "bad" type). Intermittent fasting can cause you to feel dizzy and nauseous and cause low blood sugar and dehydration periods. Although most 16:8 enthusiasts drink water during periods of fasting, it may not be enough (remember: the food itself provides quite a bit of water).

I am also much more concerned about the disordered eating behaviors that may arise as a result of intermittent fasting. Research shows that fasting for a period followed by a limited eating prime window gives you an overeat. It's a path that can be difficult to get out of because it impairs the natural hunger signals and metabolism of our body. Limited eating can also cause an increased risk of depression and anxiety.

This is particularly worrying for women, who historically were more likely to develop eating disorders. The allotted restriction periods followed by eating lend themselves to the tendencies of binge-purging that cannot (and should not) be ignored. Periods of vomiting and binging are considered risk factors for eating disorders, according to the National Eating Disorders Association.

Should you try 16:8 fasting?

It's a personal choice, in the end. But you can try some beneficial behaviors without committing to the riskier elements of 16-hour fasts. The first is to understand better the mindfulness of your food choices and how they relate to it. To begin with, put into consideration these questions when deciding on what to take:

Where are you physically when you want to eat?

Many of us feed according to situation, not greed. Case in point: if you ever went to the cinema after dinner, and suddenly wanted popcorn, raise your hand? Yeah, so do I!

You may become mindful of trends you didn't notice before by noticing the moments that you feed. Say that during The Bachelor, you are a person who loves to graze. If you're fasting at 8 p.m., you've automatically cut your post-dinner snacking hours — and then calories—short.

Are you getting enough sleep?

When you cut out snacking late-night, that alone could help you get to bed earlier— a very crucial component of any weight loss plan. Getting seven hours of sleep per night has been linked to better weight management, lowering chronic disease risk and improving metabolism.

For many of us, eliminating food to fixed periods is not feasible to achieve better health. Besides being socially challenging (who wants to skip the happy hour or dinner with friends?), self-imposed rules aren't as satisfied as having the right information and making choices that empower you versus hold you back. In the context of your daily life, it is best to find ways to make eating nutritious food work for you.

Chapter 4:

Popular Ways to Do Intermittent Fasting

Recent years have seen intermittent fasting being very trendy. It is claimed to be causing weight loss, improving metabolic health, and maybe even extending lifespan. Given the popularity, it is not shocking that several different types or methods of intermittent fasting were developed. Every method can be useful, but it depends on the individual to figure out which one works best.

Here are five standard methods to follow intermittent fasting.

1. The 16/8 Method: Fast for 16 hours each day

The 16/8 method involves fasting for 14 to 16 hours every day, and limiting your daily "eating window" to 8-10 hours. You can fit in 2, 3, or more meals within the eating window. Often known as the Leangains Protocol, this approach has been popularized by fitness expert Martin Berkhan. Merely doing this fasting process can be as easy as not eating anything after dinner and skipping breakfast. When you finish your last meal at 8 p.m., for starters, and don't eat before noon the next day, you have been fasting for 16 hours, theoretically.

It is generally recommended that women fast just 14-15 hours because, with significantly shorter fasts, they seem to do well. This approach may be hard to get used to at first for people who are getting hungry in the morning and like to eat breakfast. A lot of breakfast-skippers eat this way instinctively, though. During the fast, you can drink water, coffee, and other non-caloric drinks, which can help to reduce hunger feelings. Mostly eating healthy foods is very important during your feeding time. This method won't work if you're eating lots of junk food or too many calories.

2. The 5:2 diet: Fast for 2 days per week

The 5:2 diet involves typically eating five days a week while reducing calories to 500-600 for two days a week. This diet is also called The Easy Diet and was popularized by Michael Mosley, a British journalist. It is recommended for women to consume 500 calories on the days of fasting and for men to eat 600 calories. You would typically eat every day of the week except Mondays and Thursdays, for example. You eat two small meals for those two days (women's 250 calories per meal and men's 300 calories). No trials are evaluating the 5:2 diet itself, as the detractors correctly point out, but there is plenty of research on the effects of intermittent fasting.

3. Eat-Stop-Eat: Do a 24-hour fast, once or twice a week

Eat-Stop-Eat consists of a 24-hour fast, either once or twice a week. This method was popularized by Brad Pilon, a fitness expert, and has been popular for some years. It leads to a complete 24-hour fast by fasting from dinner one day to dinner the next. When you end dinner, for example, at 7 p.m. Monday and don't have dinner until 7 p.m. the next day, you just did a full24-hour easy. You can fast from breakfast to breakfast, or from lunch to lunch as well. The result is close.During the fast, water, coffee, and other non-caloric drinks are allowed, but no solid foods are allowed.

If you do this to lose weight, you must usually eat during the times of fasting. As in, eat the same amount of food as if you weren't fasting anyway. The potential downside of this approach is that many people may find a complete 24-hour fast relatively challenging.

You don't need to go all - in straight away, though. It's a good beginning with 14-16 hours, and then moving up from there. I have done that a couple of times myself. I found the first part of the fast very easy, but I became ravenously hungry in the last couple of hours.

To complete the full 24 hours, I needed to apply some serious self-discipline, and I often found myself giving up and eating dinner a little earlier.

4. Alternate-day fasting: Fast every other day

Alternate-day fasting means daily fasting. This approach comes in several different versions. Some of them require fasting days to be around 500 calories. Many of the laboratory studies that demonstrated the health benefits of intermittent fasting used some version of this method. Every other day, a complete fast can seem slightly extreme, so it's not recommended for beginners. With this method, several times a week, you'll be going to bed very hungry, which is not very pleasant and probably unsustainable in the long run.

5. The Warrior Diet: Fast during the day, eat a huge meal at night

The Fitness expert Ori Hofmekler popularized the Warrior Diet. During the day, it involves eating small quantities of raw fruits and vegetables and eating one massive meal at night. Basically, within a 4-hour eating window, you "fast" the entire day and "feast" the night. One of the first popular "diets" to include some form of intermittent fasting was the Warrior Diet. This diet also emphasizes food choices that are quite similar to a paleo diet — organic, unprocessed ingredients that mimic what they looked like in the wild.

With some of these approaches, a lot of people get great results. Not everybody gets intermittent fasting. It is not something that anybody has to do. It is just another tool in the toolbox that some people may find useful. Some also think women may not benefit as much as men. This may also not be a safe choice for people who have eating disorders or are susceptible to them.

If you decide to try intermittent fasting, remember to eat healthy too. During the eating periods, it is not possible to binge on junk food and expect to lose weight and improve health. Calories still count, and the quality of food is vital.

Chapter 5:

How To Do Intermittent Fasting For Weight Loss

Fasting is experiencing an increase in popularity, thanks to supporters who say that it promotes weight loss. Everyone seems to be skipping their breakfasts these days or drinking only water every third day. But is fasting healthy for you? And will it (more specifically for some) cause you to lose weight?

The short answer is yes, failure to eat can cause you to lose weight — for a while. Intermittent fasting involves a severe restriction of the intake of food for periods, which induces weight loss. It was primarily a practice associated with religious rituals or other ceremonial activities, until relatively recently. Now it is becoming a lifestyle craze in the mainstream.

If you want to lose fat, then the best strategy is intermittent fasting. Research shows that prolonged fasting — going in and out of the fasting and eating cycles — has enormous benefits for your body and mind. It can ward off chronic illness, enhance memory and brain function, and increase energy levels. What's more, intermittent fasting is an effective way to lose weight and hold it off quickly.

Intermittent fasting will easily monitor your weight loss goals by busting stubborn fat, reducing calories, and re-connecting your metabolism to improve performance. Read on for the theory behind intermittent weight loss and fasting, how to optimize your fast, and a sample routine to get you going.

Intermittent Fasting For Weight Loss

When you're fasting intermittently, you eat all the calories that your body needs but for a shorter period. There are many strategies, but feeding during a 6 to 8-hour period and fasting the remaining 14 to 16 hours is the most common method. It's not as bad as it sounds, especially if you add Coffee to keep the rates of hunger in check (more on that later).

Studies show intermittent fasting speeds up weight loss. The researchers lost a total of 10 pounds in 10 weeks in a 2015 study pooling 40 different studies. One study found that obese adults lose up to 13 pounds over eight weeks after an irregular "alternate day" fasting regimen (consuming 25 percent of their daily calories on one day, and usually eating the next day).

Intermittent fasting also succeeds where many weight-loss regimes fail: by targeting visceral fat and reducing it. Visceral fat is the rigid, tightly compressed inner fat around the abdominal organs. People on an intermittent fasting diet have been able to shed four to seven percent of their visceral fat over six months.

How Does Intermittent Fasting Boost Weight Loss?

Fasting isn't all that unusual if you think about it. Your ancestors had evolved to thrive in rare food situations. Intermittent fasting, in addition to a slew of other health benefits, causes a perfect storm of metabolic changes to combat weight loss and fat reduction. How's it making out?

How To Start Intermittent Fasting

There is no one-size-fits-all when it comes to Intermittent Fasting. Intermittent Fasting suits all your calories into 6 hours, leaving you with a daily 18-hour-fast. This is often termed fasting "18:6." Also, you can try variations like the one-meal-a-day method, or fast every other day — the trick to learning and listening to your body and seeing what works best for you. When intermittent Fasting triggers fatigue or other negative symptoms, try to fast once or twice a week, and then build up from there.

Factors to consider during your fast:

- Prospective Irritability

- Good water consumption

- Ability to differentiate between false hunger and real hunger

- Caloric deficit and resetting of the body's fat-burning hormonal environment.

- Consumption of Amino Acids during "fasting state" (specifically before and after morning "fasted state" workouts.)

Now Let's Look At The Feeding State.

This period for this day will last only the next 6-10 hours, depending on your last meal. It is advisable to consume your three main meals during this time. You still have an aka breakfast (Break the Fast) only later than the usual routine. It doesn't have to include your typical breakfast meal, but if that's your thing, it definitely can.

Every meal is going to be decent in size and will keep you going strong into the next day.

Chapter 6:

What Are The Benefits Of Eating Healthy?

A healthy diet includes a variety of multicolored fruits and vegetables, whole grains and starches, good fats and lean protein. Healthy eating often means avoiding foods, which contain high amounts of salt and sugar. We look at the top 10 advantages of a healthy diet in this review, as well as the facts behind them.

1. Weight loss

Losing weight can help minimize the risk of contracting chronic conditions. If an adult is overweight or obese, they have a higher risk of developing many diseases, including:

- non-insulin-dependent diabetes mellitus
- heart disease
- reduced bone density

Green vegetables and fruits are lower in calories than most processed foods. A person who wants to lose weight should reduce their calorie intake to not more than is needed every day. Determining the calorie requirements of an individual is simple using the dietary guidelines published by the government of the United States. Maintaining a healthy diet free of processed foods will help a person remain under their daily limits without calorie counting.

Fiber is one of the components of a healthy diet, which is especially important for weight management. Plant-based foods contain plenty of dietary fiber, helping to control appetite and making people feel fuller for longer. Researchers found in 2018 that a diet rich in fiber and lean proteins contributed to weight loss without the need for calorie counting.

2. Reduced the risk of cancer

An unhealthy diet habit can lead to obesity, which can increase the risk that a person may develop cancer. Weighing within a healthy range will lower the risk. The American Society of Clinical Oncology has been confirmed in 2014 that obesity was leading to a worse future for people with cancer. All the same, fruit and vegetable-rich diets will help protect against cancer. Researchers have found in a separate 2014 study that a fruit-rich diet reduced the risk of upper gastrointestinal tract cancers. We also observed that a diet rich in vegetables, fruits, and fiber reduced the risk of colorectal cancer and a fiber-rich diet reduced the risk of liver cancer.

Some phytochemicals found in fruits, vegetables, nuts, and legumes act as antioxidants shielding cells from cancer-causing damage. Lycopene and vitamins A, C, and E are some of these antioxidants. Human trials were inconclusive, but the findings of laboratory and animal studies linked certain antioxidants to a reduced incidence of free radical cancer-related damage.

3. Diabetes management

Eating a healthy diet will help a person with diabetes to: reduce weight, if required, maintain blood glucose levels, control blood pressure and put cholesterol levels under target limits to avoid or postpone diabetes complications. It is important for people with diabetes to restrict their consumption of foods with added sugar and salt. Also, fried foods high in saturated and trans fats are best avoided.

4. Heart health and stroke prevention

As many as 92.1 million adults in the U.S. have at least one form of cardiovascular disease according to figures released in 2017. Such disorders affect mainly the arteries of the heart or blood. According to Canada's Heart and Stroke Foundation, up to 80 percent of cases of premature heart disease and stroke can be avoided by making changes in lifestyle, such as through physical activity rates and eating healthily. There are different proof that vitamin E can prevent blood clots, which can result in heart attacks. The following foods contain high vitamin E levels: almond peanuts sunflower seeds. The medical society has long known the link between trans fats and heart-related diseases, such as coronary heart disease.

If a person excludes trans fats from the diet, this will reduce their low-density lipoprotein cholesterol levels. Another form of cholesterol causes plaque to accumulate in the arteries, which raises the risk of heart attack and stroke. Minimize blood pressure can also be essential for cardiac health, and it can help to limit salt intake to 1,500 milligrams daily. Salt is applied to many fried and fast foods and thus should be avoided by a person who wants to reduce their blood pressure.

5. The health of the next generation

Children learn from the adults around them most of the health-related behaviors, and parents who practice healthy eating habits and exercise habits tend to pass these on.

Homemade eating can also help. Researchers found in 2018 that children who often shared meals with their families consumed more greens and less sucrose food than their counterparts who eat less often at home. Additionally, children who participate in home gardening and cooking may be more likely to make healthy choices about their diet and lifestyle.

6. Strong bones and teeth

For strong bones and teeth, a diet with adequate calcium and magnesium is required. It is vital to keep the bones healthy to prevent osteoporosis and osteoarthritis later in life.

The following foods are high in calcium:

- Broccoli
- Cauliflower
- Cabbage
- Canned fish with bones
- Tofu
- Legumes

Besides, calcium fortifies certain cereals and vegetable-based milks.

In many foods, magnesium is available and the best sources are leafy green vegetables, almonds, seeds, and whole grains.

7. Better mood

Emerging evidence suggests that diet and mood are closely related. Researchers found in 2016 that a high-glycemic-loaded diet may cause increased symptoms of depression and fatigue. A high glycemic diet includes numerous refined carbohydrates, such as those found in soft drinks, cakes, white bread, and biscuits. There is a lower glycemic load of vegetables, whole fruit, and whole grains. While a healthy diet can improve general mood, seeking medical care is essential for people with depression.

8. Improved memory

A healthy diet can help prevent cognitive decline and dementia.

A 2015 report identified nutrients and foods that defend themselves against these adverse effects. We considered the following to be beneficial:

- flavonoids and polyphenols
- fish
- vitamin D, C, and E
- omega-3 fatty acids

Among other foods, the Mediterranean diet contains many of these nutritional foods.

9. Gut health Improvement

The colon is made of naturally occurring bacteria, which play significant metabolism and digestion roles. Some bacterial strains also produce vitamins K and B which support the colon. These strains also aid in the fight against bacteria and viruses particles Diet low in fiber and high in fat affects the gut microbiome, resulting in increased inflammation in the area. Diet rich in vegetables, fruits, and grains, however, provides a combination of prebiotics and probiotics that will help good colon bacteria thrive.

Fermented foods are rich in probiotics like yogurt, kimchi, sauerkraut, miso, and kefir. Fiber is a prebiotic that is easily accessible, and rich in legumes, beans, fruits, and green vegetables. Fiber also improves regular bowel movements, which can help prevent diverticulitis and bowel cancer.

10. Getting a good night's sleep

A variety of factors can disturb sleep patterns like sleep apnea. Sleep apnea happens when the airways are crossed again and again during sleep. Risk factors include obesity, alcohol consumption and eating an unhealthy diet. Reducing alcohol and caffeine consumption, whether a person has sleep apnea or not, will help to ensure restful sleep.

Quick tips for a healthful diet

There are many minor, healthy ways to improve the diet, including exchanging soft drinks for water and herbal tea without eating meat for at least 1 day a week, ensuring that intake accounts for approximately 50 percent of each meal swapping cow's milk for plant-based milk eating whole fruits instead of drinking juices that contain less fiber and often include added sugar avoiding processed meats.

A balanced diet can also be given by a doctor or dietitian.

Chapter 7:

Step-By-Step Guide to Intermittent Fasting 16/8

The 16:8 fasting program is a meal regimen in which you fast for 16 hours a day and eat in 8 hours. This diet regimen comes with all the advantages of other fasting schedules (plus, recent research has shown that it will lower blood pressure). Maybe even better, you're going to choose the food slot.

So what's the food window going to be? "There's an endless variety. It can be any day. Any moment you don't eat— that's fasting, fasting specialist, and author of The Complete Guide to Fasting. If you can't live without eating, schedule your meal early in the day (8:00 a.m. to 4:00 p.m.). If you want early dinner, eat in the middle of the day (11:00 a.m. to 6:00 p.m.).

1. Balancing the meals, no snacks between

2. Enrolling 12-12 system

3. BOOM day vol. 1

4. Enrolling 14-10 system

5. BOOM day vol. 2

6. Enrolling into the 16-8.

Balance The Meals, No Snacks Between

So when you decide to start intermittent fasting, test your previous days first. How many meals have you had?

It's all right if you don't know, if you don't remember, or if it all seemed like food all the time. That's the usual situation, as people have hectic lives nowadays.

To continue with, scatter three meals all day and don't have any snacks. Take 3 regular meals, such as breakfast, lunch, and dinner. Don't pay much attention to what you're doing, even if you're meant to get the shakes and carbohydrates out because they're going to make you want to snack and indulge once you start fasting.

Ensure you drink at least 8 cups of water a day. This process should not last more than four days, but if you need more time to adjust, that's great.

Enrolling 12-12 System

After you have learned to have two meals, it is now time to include some laws of intermittent fasting in part. Take three meals and put them in your 12 hours of food slot. And if your first breakfast is 8 a.m., your last meal should not be more than 8 p.m.

You have the sleep time in the 12-hour fasting window.

Make sure you don't eat anything 2 hours before you go to bed! You don't want to sleep after the insulin spike. Let your body accept the food you eat and slowly lower the level of insulin.

This process is estimated to be seven days max.

BOOM Day Vol. 1

Yeah, I made up this name, there's no day like BOOM.

I made that up for a reason. Just when you're happy with the system, BOOM!!! Your body doesn't like booms, even if they're safe like this one.

BOOM Day is simply a fast-extended day.

But you stick to your 12-12 schedule, and it's going to be great. You had your last dinner at 8 p.m. last night. Like you would do it every day, at 8 a.m., you're planning to break the fast. Okay, if you're all right with that, it's time for an upgrade.

Extend your pace for 8 hours.

So instead of splitting it at 8 a.m., break it down at 4 p.m. You're going to get the BOOM part now, don't you?

This isn't going to be easy, so that's what you need. It's easier to have a BOOM day, then to join a complete intermittent fasting schedule at once, and to struggle for weeks. This will cause your body to become frustrated and slip out of the comfort zone. It's going to get to the fat-burning area, and that's when the game starts.

Enrolling 14-10 System

Enrolling the 14-10 program BOOM day is over, and hopefully, you'll be able to break the 20-hour system quickly. You're going to break it now with just 10 hours to destroy the hole.

That's right, no longer than 12 hours to eat. BOOM Day will every the food window by 2 hours, which means that from now on, you're going to fast for 14 hours and eat for 10 hours.

Doing so will help you physically rebound from the BOOM day, so you certainly won't even notice that you're not eating until noon. Note, this is all about loving the process! This time should not last more than seven days.

BOOM Day Vol. 2

Here we're going again. After seven days of the 14-10 system, it's time for another BOOM day, but there's just one tiny little thing I haven't told you yet.

This BOOM day is going to last longer than the previous one. That's why he's had "vol. 2, "but that!

You're going to have to fly for 24 hours.

Surprisingly, this isn't going to be hard, as you might imagine, because you've already conditioned your body to have 0-calories-consuming times. I have fasted more than 24 hours as I did this second day of BOOM. There are two options to do this: PM.

You empty your last meal 2 hours before you leave, you don't eat anything for the whole of the next day, you go to sleep, and when you wake up in the morning, you break the fast.

I will honestly advise you to take option number 2 as the magic happens during sleep time.

As we sleep, our bodies do something like an inventory search. We take all the proteins, sugars, oils, minerals, and vitamins that we got that day, and place them where we belong. Nonetheless, if no food has been processed since the last night of sleep, our bodies will use fat to supply us with energy for the next day. You're losing weight while you're awake.

All choices will show you outcomes, but I do recommend that you take option number two.

Enrolling 16-8 System

And now you're eating intermittently!

Wooooooooooooooooooooo!

Much like the first day of BOOM, you're going to accept these opportunities a lot easier. The principle of intermittent fasting is 16-8, but it can be not very easy to achieve, and this is proved to be the easiest method I've managed to create.

In this process, you're not supposed to eat 3 hours until you sleep, and you should increase your intake of fluids.

You should stick to the 16-8 as much as you want, and even if you choose to update, you don't need to do the BOOM days anymore. Your body has become used to a broader fasting period, so you can gradually increase it.

Talking of an update, there's also an extreme variant of intermittent fasting. It's got a system of 20-4. Indeed, 20 hours of fasting and just 4 hours of food. When you want to do this, get familiar with the 16-8 system first. Push the boundaries for 1 hour if you get relaxed enough with it. You'll be astounded as the pounds fly down!

16:8 Sample Meal Plans.

Right now for the bread. Yes, 16:8 Fasting gives you the freedom to drink what you want while you're sleeping, but it's not an opportunity to go pancake-pizza-Pringles crazy.

"During your feeding times, you need to adhere to a healthy, whole food diet," says functional medicine consultant Will Cole, D.C., IFMCP, "Since some of the effects of fasting include decreased inflammation, piling on junk food during your eating cycle will exacerbate this inflammation. And with inflammation being the underlying factor leading to almost all modern-day health problems, this is something that you want to keep under control. "That means yes to protein purification, healthy fats, so carbs from whole food sources. Skip ultra-processed food and drive-thru; don't skip the emphasis on delicacies. With less time spent on food preparation and planning, it may take a lot of time.

8 a.m.: egg and veggie scramble, side of whole-grain toast

10 a.m.: yogurt and granola

12 p.m.: chicken and veggie stir fry

Evening decaf tea

Midday eating window meal plan

Morning black coffee or tea (no cream or sugar)

11 a.m.: banana peanut butter smoothie

2 p.m.: avocado toast with pistachios

4 p.m.: dark-chocolate-covered almonds

6 p.m.: turkey meatballs and tomato sauce over whole wheat (or zucchini noodle) pasta

Late eating window meal plan

Morning black coffee or tea (no cream or sugar)

1 p.m.: blackberry chia pudding

4 p.m.: black bean quesadilla (cheese of your choice, black beans, bell pepper, and taco seasoning)

6 p.m.: banana

9 p.m.: grilled salmon, vegetables, and quinoa

Chapter 8:

Benefits Of Intermittent Fasting 16/8

IF Helps You Lose Weight Without Following A Traditional, Calorie-Restricted Diet

Research suggests that counting calories and restricting food options will cause stress and increase cortisol levels, which can lead to dietary avoidance, feelings of deprivation, excessive cravings, and regaining weight. Adapting to intermittent fasting, a form of routine eating and fasting depends solely on time. Many people want more flexibility when it comes to losing weight, and they don't want to talk about dieting every day of the week, [because] they lose motivation after a certain period to reduce calories. IF works for people who like to follow the rules, instead of saying' eat less,' we advise them not to eat after 6 p.m., and for those who have the willpower, it really works.

IF Helps You Keep The Weight Off Over The Long Term

On an intermittent-fast diet, it may make it easier to sustain the weight you have gained over the period. A two-part case study of 40 obese adults, published in Frontiers in Physiology in 2016, compared the combined effects of a high-protein, low-calorie, intermittent-fast diet plan with a conventional heart-healthy diet plan. The results showed that while both diets were similarly effective in lowering body mass index (BMI) and blood lipids, those on the IF diet had a benefit in decreasing the loss of weight after one year.

IF May Help Those At Risk For Developing Diabetes

According to the United States of America. The Diseases Control and Prevention (CDC), 84.1 million people in the United States have pre-diabetes, a disease that often leads to type 2 diabetes within five years if not treated. Losing weight, exercising around, and eating a healthy diet will help prevent the development of type 2 diabetes. If you lose weight, you become more sensitive to insulin. It's pushing down the blood sugar.

As we feed, our body releases insulin into the bloodstream to provide the cells with glucose, but those who are pre-diabetes are insulin-resistant, which ensures that their blood sugar levels remain high. Intermittent fasting can benefit those who are pre-diabetic because it allows the body to produce insulin less often. If you are pre-diabetic or have a history of diabetes in your family, this type of diet may be beneficial. Evidence has shown promise in supporting these claims: a study published in the journal Cell in 2017 showed that intermittent fasting cycles could restore insulin secretion and facilitate the law of insulin beta cells in mice with type 1 and type 2 diabetes. While further work is still needed, early studies of human cell samples suggest similar promise.

IF Sync Circadian Rhythm and Shade Away Disease

The internal body clock is a natural system, which regulates sleepiness and wakefulness over a 24-hour cycle. Research published in the 2017 Annual Nutrition Review shows that intermittent fasting can help us adhere to the circadian rhythm of our body and can assist improve our metabolism. Eating these pre-bed foods has also been associated with weight gain and sleep disturbances, mainly when they induce acid reflux. We know that the sensitivity to insulin is improved during the day and that we are less sensitive to insulin at night— the same goes for digestion. This makes you wonder if having dinner at night is going against our body clock. If you want to follow the circadian rhythm, you need to go to bed earlier so that the body can heal itself.

IF May Lower Your Risk For Cardiovascular Disease

According to the CDC, approximately 610,000 people die every year of heart disease in the United States— one in every four deaths. You will reduce the risk of heart disease by adopting a healthy lifestyle: eating right, walking, not smoking, and reducing the intake of alcohol. Research also shows that intermittent fasting can benefit. This increases cardiovascular risk, glycemic control, and insulin resistance if you limit calories every day. In a small study of 32 adults published in the Nutrition Review in 2013, an alternate-day fasting regimen culminated in both weight loss and cardiovascular effects, including increased production of LDL cholesterol and triacylglycerol. Researchers use alternate-day fasting, but keep in mind that fasting doesn't mean not eating — it means eating less. That type of diet is a different way of doing things and may cater to some because they may limit a few days a week rather than every day. As an obese surgeon, I like to have a preference for patients because people are different if it is interesting to you.

Intermittent fasting Increased Growth Hormone

There are very few safe ways to improve your growth hormone levels, so fasting is just one of them. Sufficient levels of Growth Hormone (GH) mean faster regeneration, higher energy, and improved metabolism. The body also uses GH to retain proteins that protect the hair, nails, and skin.

Fortunately, not eating for a long time makes your hormone levels get a real kick. Also, these two studies (here and here) indicate that fasting will increase GH levels by between 300 and 1,205 percent.

Fasting allows you to lose weight, which automatically increases your GH. It also keeps the insulin levels under check so that it does not interfere with the development of GH.

IF May Slow Down The Aging Process

Research shows that intermittent fasting advantages can imitate the results of very-low-calorie diets that are beneficial for anti-aging. A case study published in the Journal of Cell Metabolism in 2014 showed that fasting could slow aging and help prevent and treat disease. It has been shown that fasting causes adaptive cell stress reactions, which result in a better ability to cope with more stimuli and combat disease. "Low-calorie diets improve oxidative stress, and the benefit is anti-aging. The better the mitochondria (the backbone of our cells) work, the better your body works.

IF Works Best For Certain People

Intermittent fasting may offer the greatest benefits to those who are overweight. However, people who have plateaued their weight-loss attempts may notice that intermittent fasting may help jump-start their metabolism and make them grow. It can also help those with digestive problems. Whether you find that your metabolism is late at night, or if you have digestive problems at night, feeding early and fasting overnight might help.

Often attempting a different kind of intermittent fasting is enough for some people to get back on board with their weight-loss goals. One of my nurses gained 30 pounds when she stopped eating late at night. You've got to have that "aah" for a good long-term weight loss."Time, when you remember what was the source of weight gain.

IF Can Reduce Oxidative Stress and Inflammation in The Body

Oxidative stress is one step towards aging and many chronic diseases.

This requires reactive molecules called free radicals, which interfere with and destroy other essential molecules (such as protein and DNA).

Several experiments have shown that intermittent fasting can increase the body's response to oxidative stress.

Some studies have shown that intermittent fasting can help fight inflammation, another key driver of all sorts of common diseases.

IF May be Beneficial For Heart Health

Heart disease is currently the biggest killer in the world.

It is understood that various health indicators (so-called "risk factors") are associated with an increased or decreased risk of heart disease.

Intermittent fasting has been shown to boost several different risk factors, including blood pressure, HDL and LDL cholesterol, blood triglycerides, and blood sugar levels.

Nevertheless, much of this is based on animal experiments. Effects on heart health need to be further investigated in humans before guidelines can be made.

Save A Lot Of Time (And Money)

Eating healthy requires a lot of food preparation that is very time-consuming for many people. I just view Josh Brolin being asked about his Deadpool 2 diet, and he seemed irritated that he had to feed every two hours.

By fasting, though, you save a lot of time and have more fun. Instead of cooking five to six meals a day, you can only cook one or two meals. Not will this only save you time, but you will also love what you eat a lot more as you blend your daily macros in less, but much more abundant, meals.

IF Induces Various Cellular Repair Processes

As we fly, the cells in the body start the cycle of the cell "waste removal" called autophagy.

It includes cells that break down and metabolize damaged and dysfunctional proteins that build up within cells over time.

High rate autophagy may protect against several diseases, including cancer and Alzheimer's.

IF is Good For Your Brain

What is good for the body is often useful for the brain, too.

Intermittent fasting increases the multiple metabolic characteristics considered to be essential for brain health.

It involves decreased oxidative stress, lowered inflammation, and lower blood sugar levels, and insulin resistance.

Several experiments in rats have shown that intermittent fasting may increase the growth of new nerve cells, which are supposed to improve brain function.

It also raises the levels of a brain hormone called a brain-derived neurotrophic factor (BDNF), a dysfunction that has been linked to depression and many other brain problems.

Animal studies have also shown that intermittent fasting protects against stroke injury.

IF Can Improve Your Libido.

I'm going to fully understand if you're a feminist who doesn't want more hormones in her body. But the fact is, both women and men need testosterone in their bodies because of its many advantages, especially for men.

Proper T rates will make you leaner, enhance your bone strength, and improve your libido for men. Men with high T levels typically have a high sex drive compared to men with low T levels who usually suffer from mood swings and, likely, depression. Growth Hormone often comes with a similar increase in T levels. And as intermittent fasting increases GH rates, it means that your T remains at an optimum level.

IF May Help Prevent Alzheimer's Disease

Alzheimer's disease is the most neurodegenerative disease in the world.

There is no treatment available for Alzheimer's, so stopping it from occurring in the first place is essential.

Research in rats showed that intermittent fasting could delay the onset of Alzheimer's disease or reduce its severity.

In a variety of case reports, dietary therapy requiring regular short-term rapids was able to significantly improve Alzheimer's symptoms across 9 out of 10 cases.

Animal studies also indicate that fasting can protect against other neurodegenerative diseases, including Parkinson's and Huntington's.

IF May Cure Fatty Livers

Fatty liver happens as fat is more than 5% to 10% of the weight of your liver. This occurs to heavy drinkers and overweight people when the body is unable to metabolize fat fast enough and, if left untreated, the fatty liver will turn into cirrhosis.

What does fasting sell the fatty liver to you?

According to a 2016 case study by the German Environmental Health Research Centre, fasting helps the liver give a protein called GADD45b (Growth Arrest and DNA Damage-inducible) responsible for regulating the synthesis of fatty acids in the liver. The increase in this GADD45b protein in your body normalizes the fat content of the liver and decreases the amount of sugar in your blood.

IF May Extend Your Lifespan, Helping You Live Longer

One of the most promising aspects of intermittent fasting may be its potential to prolong the lifetime.

Studies in rodents have shown that intermittent fasting increases lifespan in the same manner as constant calorie restriction.

In some of these trials, the results have been quite drastic. In one of them, the rats who fasted every other day lived 83 percent longer than the rats who did not fast.

While this is far from established in humans, intermittent fasting has become very common among the anti-aging crowd.

Given the known effects of metabolism and all sorts of health markers, it makes sense that intermittent fasting will help you live longer and healthier lives.

Chapter 9:

Potential Mistake And Downside Of

Intermittent Fasting 16/8

A lot of people are looking to lose weight. Fasting, voluntary abstention from food, is a common form of weight loss with a long record of success. Nonetheless, many people forget about the cardinal rule of Fasting, or indeed about any dietary change–make sure you do it safely.

But, taken to extremes, Fasting can also have its risks. This is valid not only for Fasting but for anything. When you take veganism to heights, you may be at risk of vitamin B12 deficiency, for example. When you make a low-fat diet to extremes, you are at risk of vitamin D deficiency. When you take the salt limitation to limits, you may be at risk of quantity depletion. When you take extreme activity, you may be at risk for muscle breakdown. must be done responsibly, with knowledge and common sense.

Fasting isn't any different. Since Fasting is already more rigorous than most diets, bringing Fasting to extremes can be troublesome. The film explores some of the risks of Fasting and examines many of the fasting alternatives that are common and may be beneficial to people. Simply put, Fasting is a tool to be used in the fight against obesity-related conditions and perhaps some age-related conditions.

But, like any knife, it's got two sides. It has potential power, and that power can be used constructively, and it can also be used destructively in the wrong hands. It's all a matter of applicability. Most of the resurgence of interest in fasting as a therapeutic alternative revolves on intermittent Fasting—generally shorter duration, regularly and often. The 5:2 diet is two days of Fasting per week, but the fasting days only require 500 calories per day. A time-limited diet, such as a 16:8 regimen, requires you to eat just 8 hours a day so that 16 hours of Fasting is expended. A lot of24-hour to 36-hour fasts 2-3 days a week, and this is performed under medical supervision with your doctor.

For example, I also use prolonged Fasting, but generally limited to 7-14 days, only in the appropriate person and under observation. Longer speeds have more power, but more risk. To me, there is no reason to run to 30 consecutive days just for the sake of contention. Why not make 4 different 7-day fasts instead? It will have roughly the same positive health effects with a much lower risk.

In Fasting, on the other side, there was a young lady who decided to join a 30-day water-only fasting retreat. As far as I can say, there was no medical monitoring, and there were no blood tests being reviewed, and there was no specialist who even decided whether it was necessary. One of my crucial fasting principles is that if someone is underweight or is worried about malnutrition, they shouldn't be easy. Underweight is characterized by the Body Mass Index < 18.5, but for a safety margin, I do not recommend that anyone be fast more than 24 hours if they have a BMI < 20. The logic seems quite clear. During the fasting period, the body must withstand the accumulation of nutrients and energy. If you have an excess of body fat (stored food energy), then you should be fine. If you don't have a lot of body fat, then it's not all that. It's dumb, man.

Citizens get into trouble with deep rapids because they don't practice common sense. Many of these fasting retreats give only fasts for 30 days of water. If you become sodium-depleted (very common), there are no doctors there to check for warning signs. If you become exhausted and unable to get out of bed, there is something wrong, and you should not carry on Fasting. Okay, that's common sense. With my IDM system, people know that they may feel hungry, maybe a little irritable, constipated, but they shouldn't feel UNWELL. If you really feel bad, you've got to stop. There is no need to go on because Fasting is easy. It's much better to stop and try again (if you want) in a couple of days when you're feeling better. The issue with these fasting retreats is that people have paid money to be there and are therefore going far beyond the boundaries of good safety practice and far beyond the limits of common sense.

Therefore, people practice intense Fasting without any planning. Instead of pursuing shorter speeds and slowly extending them, they quickly opted for a complete water-only extended rate. It's like an inexperienced mountaineer who wants to attempt Mount Everest, without oxygen and drive it to the summit, whatever the conditions. The seasoned mountaineer will immediately recognize this as a wish to die, but the novice has no inkling of the risks and may come home in a body bag. It's a pure stupid thing. But fasting hospitals are spreading the same notion. Take the most severe fast (water-only Fasting, as opposed to allowing any bone marrow or caloric intake) for an extended period (30 days instead of 1-2 days) in anyone, irrespective of whether this is medically appropriate, without adequate medical monitoring or access to blood work? For now, I can assure you, that's pure stupidity.

Call the marathon story. According to myth, in 490 BC, the Greek hero Pheidippides raced about 26 miles from the frontline near the town of Marathon to Athens to send news of the defeat of the Persians. He roared at Niki! (Victory) and then he knelt instantly and collapsed.

Suppose a sedentary, middle-aged, out-of-shape guy decided to run 26 miles at maximum speed tomorrow, without any kind of planning or awareness. He could keel over and die, too. Nonetheless, in 2014, a 42-year-old man died after the London Marathon, the second death of the race in three years. Earlier that year, a 31-year-old man and a 35-year-old man died in North Carolina. Because the marathon is a relatively extreme occurrence for most people, it takes some planning to be done safely. That's easy to understand, but you can't see the hysteric headlines saying, "Playing, the riskiest thing ever." If you want to hide for a few minutes, you certainly won't be killed. Running a marathon in a new state could do that very well.

The bottom line, though, is that Fasting, done correctly and with knowledge, is an effective factor in the fight against diseases and obesity. Yet devices can cut both ways, and they can sometimes damage the user. A chainsaw is a powerful tool to cut branches. It can also kill you if it is misused. But the right lesson is not to leave the chainsaw. Alternatively, we need to know how to use the tool properly. Fasting used safely, maybe a powerful force for wellbeing. Fasting, misused, will hurt or kill you — fasting by beginning to skip a meal here and there–a good idea. Fasting by beginning 30 days without water is quickly approaching hell or high water–a bad idea.

Chances are, you've come to this book because you're having trouble with your fast — you're not seeing the weight come off, your appetite isn't improving, and you're depressed for most hours of the day.

We're going to dive into the most common intermittent fasting errors you're likely to make and how to correct them.

Intermittent Fasting (IMF) is not a diet, and it is a method of feeding. Most specifically, this is a way of life. It doesn't have anything to partaking with the food you should consume, but when you have this. Relatively simple and straightforward, the 16/8 approach is the most common way to achieve sporadic rpm. It includes skipping breakfast and feeding only in the 8-hour duration of the day while fasting for the other 16.

Since intermittent fasting does not lead to extensive research, it is difficult to provide conclusive evidence. Remember the end goal of improving the body's structure and giving it a standard refresh every day. IF is by no means a one-size-fits-all lifestyle. But it's worth a try!

Overeating

This is one of, if not the most essential, intermittent fasting errors that we see people making as they start implementing the IMF. If you don't consume a healthy amount of food while you're sleeping, that can make you feel thirsty for AF while you're quick, in effect, leading you to overeat right at noon. Have you been going overboard? Chances are you've been sabotaging your rhythm (and your metabolism) along with it.

Overeating is mainly due to our emotional response to fasting. In a world where food is available at our disposal, readily available in our refrigerators, and with a click of a button shipped to our house, we're used to seeing food all the time. If you run, the brain thinks differently, and when you stop eating, it tricks you into believing that you have to eat as much of you as you can in a state of starvation. This is called binging, too.

Say you're used to consuming 2,000 calories a day, and you're starting to fly. You're going for 12-16 hours without eating, you've had your first bite of food at 11 a.m., and the next thing, you've lost your lunch and your best friends, and you can't satisfy that appetite. You're eating so much, you don't want to feed again (like any little meals in the afternoon), and you're eating another big dinner because you're feeling so thirsty when you're out of college. Next thing you know, by the end of the day, you've eaten two huge meals consisting of 3,000 calories and the start of your next easy. You feel like crap, you sleep like garbage, and you can't eat anything for the next 12 hours. See the spiritual environment that you just poured yourself into?

Take it easy on your carbs, pal. My advice is to eat 2-3 medium-sized meals in your fast and have a healthy snack or two in-between. Program your brain, and your body will obey.

Under-eating

Calorie reduction is an efficient way to lose weight, but it can lead to unintended effects when combined with intermittent fasting. It leads to under-eating during your 8-hour period, and if you're under-eating and high, your body can fail, hang on to body fat, and actively try to get rid of muscle. Yes! Yeah! Think about the opposite effect you're going to have, huh?

For short, if you don't eat plenty, you're going to gain weight. Fasting is going against the natural physical cues (like appetite or fullness), so it's essential to understand how much (and what) you need to consume while you're fasting. The best way to do that? Getting a diet consultant, help you out and develop a plan that fits your desires and expectations when it comes to your intermittent fasting and body goals.

Eating too early

You want to deplete as much glycogen as you can all day, so that means you'll move your meal window until later in the day. How can that help you? Okay, let's look at an example of this. Think the fasting time is 4 p.m. It's at 8 a.m. And your breakfast time is 8 a.m. Around four o'clock.

As a general guideline, it takes from 6 and 12 hours for your body to get into a rapid state after you've stopped eating, based on what you've already eaten. So at least your body uses glycogen stores for 4 hours after your last meal. But at the moment, you're unconscious.

You're not running around or working out, so you're not using as much glycogen as you could because your body isn't involved. And after you wake up at 8 a.m. You break your fast and your insulin spikes that stop the process of fat burning.

What I recommend is that you have your last meal just before you go to bed. Let's take a look at another example: the fasting time is from 11 p.m. Up to 3 p.m. And the mealtime is 3 p.m. Around 11 p.m. And you're enjoying your last dinner at 10:30 p.m.

While you're asleep, your body is going into a strong rhythm, and by the time you wake up at 8 a.m. You're more than halfway there already.

So, all day long, you're driving, taking the stairs, working out, and just going about your day, and your body is using glycogen stored in your fat cells. By the time you hit your pace at 3 p.m., You helped burn some of the fat in your body.

The Fast Doesn't Work Without The Feast

Fasting is not a magic pill or magic at all. One of the most significant intermittent fasting errors you could make? Ignoring what you eat for the sake of food.

Yeah, we get it, changing habits is challenging, but if you're not willing to improve what you're eating, including enjoying the processed food single pack burritos from the frozen section instead of some oatmeal or eggs and bacon in the morning, then what? Intermittent fasting is probably not going to work for you, and no other diet is going to work until you are genuinely ready to change from eating processed foods to whole foods.

If you forget what you're drinking, this intermittent fasting error is compounded by some significant drawbacks. We're worried about muscle loss, increased body fat, reduced weight loss, and a serious lack of nutrients. You're fasting now, so why make it harder for your body?

Make sure you choose the most nutrient-dense, nourishing food for the celebration process of your day. It contains beef, balanced carbs, healthy fats, and fruit. The better you do this part, the better you're going to make it through your fast without being too hungry or undernourished.

Drinking The Wrong Thing During The Fast

What do you have to drink during intermittent fasting? Great question, guy! Reports are coming out lately that provide users with more statistical evidence that supports what you can and can not drink, but at this moment, the more comfortable you can handle what you drink, the healthier.

Sources of what you can drink during intermittent fasting include:

- Purified Water or Electrolyte Water
- Baking Soda & Water
- Water &Glauber's Salt
- Herbal Teas
- Black Coffee
- Apple Cider Vinegar

- Fasted Lemon & Cayenne Pepper Water

What are you not supposed to drink during your sporadic fast? As a general rule of thumb, you can stay away from sweetener drinks because they will allow the body to respond to insulin (precisely what we're trying to keep away from in a fasted state).

All in all, try not to drink anything with a caloric benefit or anything that will raise the insulin. Avoid this intermittent fasting error and continue in your fast, longer time to reap more benefits.

Many people will argue that, for example, caffeine or lemon water would kill you quickly. Since there is inconclusive evidence and there are several explanations for fasting, we recommend doing what's best for you and your priorities.

You Aren't Moving Your Body

Listen, I think the war is all right. There are people in the world who enjoy gyms. We enjoy sweat and exercise, that's their stuff. And then there are people in the world like me who need a solid kick in the back to get them out for a 20-minute walk.

The bottom line is that if you don't workout or keep your body healthy, you won't grant yourself the best chance of success in the regimen.

As you exercise, you help your body get faster, and you help it deplete its glycogen stores quicker, because when you workout, the body's primary energy supply is glycogen. This is a great reason why you should do your best to work out before you break down easily and even more if you workout in the morning.

Nonetheless, this is not the only alternative. Working out, in general, is good for your health. Yet working out in a fasted state is perfect for losing fat.

Also, you need to find out if you want to see the weight and lack of fat. When you work out before your body reaches a fasted state, you help your body get further into a fasted state by depleting glycogen.

If you're operating in a fasted state, you're making the body burn the glycogen in your fat cells.

IMF Doesn't Fit Your Lifestyle

If the key doesn't suit, why are you still trying to jam it in the door? Intermittent fasting isn't for everyone, despite all the hype, and if you've tried it, and you've done everything you can to make it a success, and you're still having problems, it's all right to get away from it. When you love food, and it's your favorite meal of the day, because it gives you the strength you need to improve your day, then keep on eating it. If you're an athlete who starts at 5 a.m. and squirts on an empty stomach, then' grab the Tina stuff' and go exercise. When you work the night shift, and fasting gives you a significant energy loss, don't do it.

Often we try so hard to achieve our goals that we risk our overall health. This may include your financial, physical, or emotional health. If the IMF doesn't work for you, or even if it does, the most effective way to make a difference in your wellbeing is by eating whole, healthy, and natural foods.

On the other hand, if you try the IMF and it's hard for you because you're starving and don't get where you want to go as soon, give it more than a week or two. Studies show that it takes 28 days to make a pattern stick, and if you're trying to make IF work for you, skip these typical intermittent fasting errors and give it your best shot.

If you want to lose more weight, improve your appetite, and improve your overall health, intermittent fasting can be an excellent option for you, your goals, and your lifestyle. When you find yourself following all the rules, and you don't like them, so know it's just not for you and move on. Our best recommendation is this: listen to your body and be in touch with what you're trying to tell you, not just what you've read online, what some people have said, or what a company is trying to offer you.

Chapter 10:

Dangers Of Intermittent Fasting 16/8

There's some evidence to back it up. A case study published in the journal Obesity showed that participants eat by 8 a.m. And at 2 p.m. We had smaller appetites and less body fat.

Nevertheless, like any diet, intermittent fasting can lead to extreme eating habits.

In some cases, the adverse side effects of fasting may outweigh any potential benefits.

If you're always worried about what to eat next, it could be a sign of orthorexia.

Dieting, in general, can lead to orthorexia, a condition that includes an obsession with healthy eating. Some of the symptoms of orthorexia show the need to think about your food all the time and stress about your next meal.

One of the overarching signs is when the diet starts to become unyielding. It means changing or canceling social outings because they don't suit the eating habits.

Intermittent fasting can disrupt your sleep, which is critical to health.

There is some preliminary evidence that overnight fasting will enhance sleep by preventing you from waking up in the middle of the night. If people start fast early, their food window often begins to close just before they go to bed. It helps them avoid overnight snacks that can improve the quality of their sleep.

Intermittent fasting can also interrupt the sleep cycle or lead to restless nights. Multiple studies have shown that fasting will reduce the amount of REM sleep that is assumed to improve memory, mood, and cognitive ability.

It could also make you less aware.

Intermittent fasting may contribute to diminished alertness, as the body does not eat enough calories during a fasting period to provide enough strength. Fasting could also lead to exhaustion, difficulties in focusing, or dizziness.

Your diet shouldn't include self-shaming.

If people give themselves a window of time to eat, they will begin to feel bad for breaking their fast too early or eating too late, Rumsey said. Any fear or embarrassment about your diet can be a warning sign of dysfunctional behavior, she said. It involves thinking to yourself when you're waiting for another symptom of orthorexia.

IF can increase levels of cortisol, making you stressed.

Early research has shown that intermittent fasting can reduce the risk of diabetes, obesity, and heart disease, which can lead to increased levels of cortisol, the body's stress hormone, being deprived of food for a more extended period.

Even if there are theoretically any positive health effects, the rise in tension will counteract them.

If you lose your period, it could be related to fasting.

Intermittent fasting can lead to a calorie deficit in some cases, which can lead to hair loss and prolonged or missing hours. Those on an intermittent fasting diet may also feel colder than usual due to low blood sugar levels.

Anxiety and depression could be a tip-off that your diet isn't healthy.

Intermittent fasting leads to disordered feeding when it begins to affect one's health. It involves a difference in mental and social activity, such as a rise in anxiety and depression.

If you feel "hangry," you might want to consider putting a stop.

We've just got a natural night quick while we sleep. Normally, I don't advocate any kind of strict fasting outside of that, because what you're doing is suppressing your body's instincts.

Instead, people should listen to their body's natural cues as to whether they're hungry or finished.

Getting hungry is a real thing to do. Individuals can get irritable.

Avoid Fasting If You Have Higher Caloric

Individuals who are underweight, dealing with weight gain, under 18 years of age, pregnant or breastfeeding should not attempt an intermittent fasting diet because they need sufficient calories daily to develop appropriately.

You should stop fasting entirely if you are at risk of eating disorders. Intermittent fasting has a strong correlation with bulimia nervosa, and, as a result, people who are vulnerable to eating disorders should not undergo fasting-related diets. Risk factors for eating disorders include having someone suffering from an eating disorder, perfectionism, impulsivity, and mood disturbance.

You will most likely feel bloated, overeat, dehydrated, exhausted, and irritable. Intermittent fasting is not for the faintness of your spirit, which means if you are not underweight, you are over 18 years, you are not predisposed to eating disorders, and you are not a pregnant or breastfeeding mother, you will most likely have some unwanted side effects.

You will most likely notice that your stomach crumbles during fasting times, mainly if you are used to frequent grazing throughout the day. To prevent these hunger pains during fasting cycles, avoid looking at, tasting, or even thinking about food that can cause the secretion of gastric acid into your stomach and make you feel thirsty.

Non-fast days are not days when you can splurge on whatever you want, as this can lead to weight gain. Fasting can also lead to a high rate in the stress hormone which can lead to even more food cravings. Keep in mind that over-eating and binge eating are two common side effects of intermittent fasting.

Intermittent fasting is sometimes correlated with dehydration because when you don't sleep, you often fail to drink, so it's important to stay adequately hydrated throughout the day through consuming, on average, three liters of water.

You're more likely to feel exhausted because your body is running on less energy than usual, and because fasting will raise stress levels, it can also interrupt your sleep patterns. It is, therefore, essential to follow a safe, regular sleep schedule and adhere to it so that you can feel refreshed daily.

The same biochemistry that controls mood also influences appetite with food intake affecting the function of neurotransmitters such as dopamine and serotonin, which play a role in anxiety and depression.

This means which deregulating your appetite may do the same to your mood, so you're more likely to feel irritable when you're fasting.

The last piece of advice for people who are involved in an intermittent fasting diet is that the consumption of alcohol is reduced only during feeding times. Do not drink alcohol during or shortly after fasting, and even if you drink during your feeding times, keep in mind that drinking alcohol means that you are displacing the potential for adequate nutrition.

Chapter 11:

Tips And Hack To Success Of Intermittent Fasting 16/8

Intermittent fasting, also shortened to "IF," can be a highly effective means of weight loss. However, contrary to what some people say, it is not a form of hunger or poverty. Speak of intermittent fasting more like time-controlled feeding. It doesn't have to be focused on when you don't feed (like starvation), but instead when you do.

Here are some great tips and tricks that will help you adhere to your intermittent fasting goals. These are strategies that are all easy to implement, produce impressive results, and make the diet plan simpler.

Use the method that works for you

There are three main types of intermittent fasting: fasting for 24 hours, once or twice a week, and daily food on the other days.

Eat all of your calories within 8 hours and fast for the other 16 hours of the day.

Restricted calories 1-2 days a week with healthy food for the remaining five days, typically 500-600 calories on restricted days.

Several variables help you determine which form of intermittent fasting would work best for you. Are you an early bird, huh? Should you work a lot of hours? Are you single or have a partner that will be influenced by your eating habits?

Don't panic if it takes a few attempts to find the program that best suits you. The purpose of the IF is to help you live your best life. It can only do it for you if you hold to the program to make your life better, not more burdensome. It's all right to change the feeding schedule while you're fasting intermittently, the important thing is to find the system that works for you. Experimentation is a good thing!

Stay Hydrated!

Water is a vital part of staying alive, and it's especially important when you're fasting. Drinking water regularly all day will not only save you from getting so thirsty, but it will also keep your organs occupied.

Did you know that many times people make a hunger error for starvation? A little desire that creeps through you, dryness in your throat, and a little touch of irritation? This is hunger more often than you would think. If you can drink cold water or ice water, the cold will refresh you more than lukewarm or room temperature water, and it will give your stomach a little shock that will quench your hunger for longer.

Drink at least 64 oz of water a day. When you work out regularly, you'll need more water. Make sure you drink at least a full glass of water before and after your workout, mainly if you can't or don't like to drink water during your workout.

Buy a bottle of water that can hold at least 16 oz of water. You'll need to refill at least four times a day to get your 64 oz, but sometimes emptying and refilling can be a fun challenge. You can gamify the game by giving yourself time limits to drinking each round, or by giving yourself little incentive when you hit your quota early.

Find your unique cycle

Whenever necessary, avoid eating 2-3 hours before you go to bed, but everything else is up to you. It's normal to continue a quick, 24-hour dinner and breakfast with dinner the next night, but it doesn't have to be that way.

If you're an early morning runner or a gym rat, you could get your exercise, eat breakfast, and then track your start time. And, if you've got a hectic work schedule that's especially crazy on a few days of the week, you could have a quick time around the days you can have lunch.

The same principle applies to limited consumption days or8-hour time restrictions. Do not try to force your identity into a structure that is unpleasant or painful.

Don't Rush Yourself

It always takes time to get used to something different, no matter how excited you are or how much you want it to work for you. That definition may be more accurate to our eating habits than to anything else in our lives.

The way we eat is often rooted in us since we are young. Conscious intermittent fasting is not something that our parents teach most of us. It's a process that we learn as adults, even after the complexities of our eating habits have been cemented.

What does it all mean? Beginning Intermittent Fasting is a massive change for you— physically, spiritually, psychologically. It's all right to take it slow and be flexible. Give yourself a break, please!

It is not expected that new drivers will hop into the vehicle and get straight on the highway. Set realistic goals for yourself and let yourself have a learning curve. That's the only way your experiment of Intermittent Fasting can end up as a safe, balanced eating habit.

Hunger Pains? Create a Diversion.

Sometimes the pain of starvation can be severe during intermittent fasting. They will stop you from work or deter you from doing company. An easy and effective way to fight these hunger pains is to create a diversion for your stomach. (2) Make yourself a cup of hot tea— herbal or caffeine, depending on where you're in your day and what you're up to. Tea has almost no calories in it (as long as you don't pour milk or sugar in it), but it will warm your body and fill your stomach. Caffeinated black or green tea is a great way to give you a little lift and concentrate on it. Herbal tea is going to soothe and calm you as you start to wind your day.

Think ahead to your fast break meal – plan it out.

The best thing you can do for yourself with intermittent fasting, especially at the beginning, is to plan your fast-breaking meal. You're likely to feel very hungry the first few times you stick to quick, healthy, in a way you might not have felt before. Planning your fast-breaking lunch ahead of time will help keep you in control of your appetite.

Traps planning will help you avoid the following:

- **Emotional eating:** You're not going to grab the first enticing junk food you see. Keeping junk food out of your home will help you avoid eating physically, but don't feel like you need to hide indoors! There are fast food places all over the world these days, and the temptations to eat are limitless. Let your meal plan keep you focused on target and light.

- **Overeating:** You're going to be less likely to feed with your head and take extra portions that you don't need. Hunger informs the brain that it has to stock up on food if there is another long wait before food is available again. That reflex is a powerful instinct from when humans had to hunt for food and cook, and no food was assured. Preparing your fast-breaking lunch as thoroughly as possible will prevent you from sinking into an ancient desire to eat as much as possible.

- **Psyching yourself out:** Even when it's time to tick, it can feel like it's forever until your next meal during intermittent fasting. But if you know exactly what you're going to do before your tempo is over, you're going to have a much better target. It's going to give you warmth and relieve your innate insecurity about your appetite. We are often our own worst enemy when it comes to the way we eat. There are a thousand different ways to kill yourself when the tempo comes to an end. Providing a simple, easy-to-achieve meal plan for your quick will give you the support you need to stay on the right track.

Eat Heartily: Give Your Stomach Work

The easiest way to keep the hunger pain away is to give your stomach a lot of work to do. Think of your stomach as an active child. The more exciting and stimulating an experience you can give the kid, the more it's functioning and not looking for something else to do. A precocious child can cause a lot of damage in a short period if left unfulfilled. Say that your stomach is the same way—it's left without food to digest, to keep it occupied, it's going to start pestering you for something to do. The longer your stomach sits, the heavier your appetite is, and the worse the hunger pains become.

Keep away from light, airy foods during your last meal before you start a quick snack. You want to eat foods that have real substance to them. We're not thinking about heavy things like cake and pie (although they're good as mild treats), but rather about nutritious foods that your stomach will need to work to break down.

Consider the following types of food:

- **Leafy vegetables** like spinach, broccoli, chard, and dark lettuces.
- **Potatoes** with the skins on; roasting helps keep the most nutrients in.
- **Grains** like brown rice, wheat pasta, and oatmeal.
- **Soups** that combine many of the ingredients above; but be careful – store-bought soups are often loaded with sodium and processed meat.
- **Fruits** that will give you energy like bananas, apples, grapes, and oranges.

Fasting Doesn't Mean Sitting Around

A lot of people are afraid to go out into the world while they're on the hard. There are endless temptations beyond your house. It could be a challenging idea to go out and meet them while you're fasting.

Yet locking yourself inside is not going to help you in the long run. Not only does it push you to feel lonely and isolated, but it could also make you hate fasting for making you stay inside or unwittingly develop a new bad habit that makes you afraid to eat outside your house.

Go out there and live your life! If it's supposed to be a different part of your life, not to deter you from enjoying it. Select places where the temptations may be less or less tempting to you. Bring friends and help for you.

Eat Foods You Love

This trick is the second most important because it's so important not to forget that you're doing Intermittent Fasting to make you feel better. It's supposed to be a happy and pleasant trip, not an endless method of torture.

Intermittent fasting doesn't tell you what you can and can't eat. This makes you know when to eat and at what pace. Of course, eating healthy and nutritious meals will help you lose weight sooner and more quickly, but that doesn't mean you need to eat healthy foods that you dislike.

Your feeding times will feel much more regular and smoother once you stop fasting with food that you enjoy eating. Not a fruit addict, huh? There's no question! Don't you like to eat meat? Get your protein somewhere else.

Water intake is extremely important.

One of the essential factors in any diet plan is to ensure that your body is well hydrated. By actually drinking a glass of water before each meal, the water can reduce your hunger and make you feel better (so you can stop overeating). Water is going to wash out all the toxins, and the hunger level is going to be much lower.

Listen to Your Body

This is the most critical hack of all— it's your "SELF" hack. React to what the body is telling you to do. It's essential to find and stick to a program, but it's not worth physical or emotional pain.

Intermittent fasting is all about motivating yourself to take control of the way you eat. This ensures that you have full permission to make a shift if it's not going well.

Perhaps one day, 24 hours before you need to eat it, you don't make it completely. When 22 o'clock rolls around and your body begs you to feed—it's all right! Don't beat yourself up, man. Make a healthy choice — slice the cucumber, eat the peach, and have a bowl of oatmeal. Decompress, let go of it, and keep moving.

Intermittent Fasting Frequency

There is no appropriate or incorrect solution to an intermittent fasting schedule— there is only a schedule that works best for you. Keep a close eye on your strength, attitude, and weight loss success, observing how various methods impact you physically and mentally.

Many people practice intermittent fasting on a weekly or bi-weekly basis to make the most of the benefits. Below are a couple of fasting plans that might work for you.

Those who observe intermittent fasting daily will typically have a shorter fasting time and a more extended feeding period. Of starters, if you adopt the 16/8 form of intermittent fasting, you can skip breakfast every day, becoming your first meal of the day.

Weekly Fasts

If you choose a fasting window that lasts 24 hours or longer, it is recommended that you only practice intermittent fasting 1–2 times a week. Fasting is more rational than it could cause muscle loss or other adverse effects.

Bi-Weekly Fasts

If your fast lasts 36 or 48 hours, it's best to take a full week or two weeks off between fasts. Start with a more moderate approach, taking two full weeks off between rapids. When the body is more used to training, you should plan for a more aggressive approach, with just one week off in between.

Skipping Meals

If you're new to intermittent fasting and everyday worries you, missing food is a useful shortcut. If you're eating a big meal, try skipping coffee. If you're busy at noon, skip lunch and have an early dinner.

Although conventional wisdom once cautioned that it would never miss food and mark breakfast as the "most important meal of the day," new research contradicts these views. Skipping food will improve your metabolism, not inhibit it. It seems that skipping breakfast might be just as good as skipping dinner, so take your pick.

If you miss one meal, be careful not to overeat the next. The aim of losing food is to become an intelligent eater — to consume only when you're hungry, not because it's "the time" to enjoy a meal. It's not a reason to gorge on your next sit-down lunch or pursue other types of eating disorders.

Skipping Meals Schedule

If you choose to skip meals instead of keeping to a daily fasting schedule, your eating routine could look different every day of the week. Start by missing a meal when you're not hungry, then try to miss a few meals spaced throughout the week.

- Skip breakfast: Eat only lunch and dinner.

- Skip lunch: Eat breakfast, fast throughout the workday, then eat dinner.

- Skip dinner: Enjoy breakfast and lunch, then do an overnight fast.

Chapter 12:

How To Get Motivated

Motivation is what pushes us to make things happen—but keeping motivated is not always straightforward. Motivation is what moves you towards a mission, gets you up in the morning, and keeps you going through a job that is resolved to achieve when things get tough. Nevertheless, inspiration can be both positive and negative:

- Good motives rely on the good things that will happen as you take action. For starters,' Finishing this task means I'm just a step away from being eligible.'

- Negative motives rely on the negative backlash that will result if you don't take action. For example:' If I don't complete this assignment in the next few hours, I'm going to fail my test.

Both negative and positive motives can be successful in different circumstances. It's much better to do something, though, if you want to do it, rather than because you want to stop a particular outcome if you don't. If you don't have an affirmative action plan, using constructive reinforcement will make you feel powerless and can decrease your motivation. Regardless matter what you're focused on, there's going to be days when you don't feel like showing up. There's going to be exercises you don't feel like having. There are rumors that you don't feel like publishing. There's going to be tasks that you don't feel like doing. And there will be "bad days" where the energies then feelings are in the gutter. Those changes are part of life, and I have to face those emotional struggles just as much as the next person. Nonetheless, I have also developed a system for coping with these "bad days" for the essential things in my life.

HOW TO GET MOTIVATED ON 3 DAYS INTERMITTENT FASTING 16/8

3 Day Intermittent Fast, Day 0

Last Meal

To toast (Mourn?), I had a beautiful and humongous Sunday night meal with some Toblerone and a drink to enjoy. Then I started my 3 days strong. No more frying, cooking, or eating for 72 hours. It's just juice, tea, lemon, and black coffee.

I went to sleep feeling like a marathoner is about to launch his first run.

3 Day Intermittent Fast, Day 1

Setting Off on a Voyage of Self-Discovery

My first day was kind of like that of an early adventurer searching for the New World. I wasn't entering new territory— I'd done fasts 24 hours before — but this time it was different. I didn't turn back this time. I felt anxious and nervous.

Monday morning began with my regular heavy lifting workout at the gym (and a new personal best!), followed by a lot of online computer work.

Things got strange, then.

Something's Missing

Usually, I should have had a large breakfast early in the afternoon, but this time, nothing. It's all black coffee.

That was worse than not to eat was not to have a daily lunch break for me. Instead of catching up on sports and social media while slurping down a smoothie and some bacon, I just kept working. Who would have thought that fasting could lead to more productivity? Surprise!

My girlfriend Kim, who was supposed to be out until Thursday, shocked me by coming home early. And since I didn't tell her about my 3-day quick strategy, she had brought some fresh salmon for dinner. Wow. Damn.

Surprisingly though, even as I watched and tasted her cook and eat her delicious-looking food with lust, I didn't feel hungry. I was feeling good.

3 Day Intermittent Fast, Day 2

Uncharted Territory

What a strange feeling it is to wake up for the first time in my life after a day of zero calories. I may joke that I felt hollow inside, but I didn't think so. I was feeling great. My sleep-tracking ring even said that my sleep quality was 95%.

Feeling Electric From the beginning of day 2 to the conclusion of my 3-day fast, my mind felt electrical. As if I was high on Adderall, I didn't feel so centered in years.

It, I found out later when I read some books on the biology of fasting, is complete to be expected. My brain was running on better gasoline than it used to, and my whole body benefited from hormone boosts.

I worked in a hyper-focused environment all morning. So, when my eyes began to twitch from staring too much at the phone, I went to the nearby beach to unwind. I've been trying to meditate for 20 minutes, and holy hell! At a certain level, I swear to God that I felt heavy. It's incredible.

The First Poor Experience Like Day 1, I certainly didn't make any personal bests in my Day 2 exercise. I felt like I did the day I tried to work out after I took a bus from Lima to Huaraz in Peru (3000 meters or 10,000 feet).

My body felt good, but it didn't have the stamina it usually did. Between one or two lifts, my energy evaporated, and sometimes I became lightheaded to the point of dizziness.

I was happy I had some exercise, but it was the first negative effect I experienced during my three days.

Unusual Day Again, it was a ride not to have my daily food brakes for lunch and dinner. I missed the ritual more than the food itself. I didn't know what I had to do with myself. It was like a double daylight saving time: usually at 11 p.m. I'm ready for bed, but this time I was prepared by 9 p.m. My brain wasn't going to stop humming, though, so I ended up reading in bed for hours.

Oh yeah, and most critically (and disappointingly): no garbage. No number two at all on Day two of my three days fast.

3 Day Fast, Day 3

What the Hell?

Generally, I wake up at 7:15 a.m. Tomorrow, huh? I was up at 5 a.m. and ready to go. My sleep-tracking ring told me that I had a 90% sleep quality.

I wasn't hungry yet, and my mind was sharp. So did my hearing and my sense of smell, which seemed oddly super-powerful. However, my body felt lethargic.

The strangest thought, though? It's my head.

My mouth was like a warehouse in a business that had just gone bankrupt. It's all spice and stretch, and it's ready to go, but it's bare. My air felt oddly new and flat, and my mouth was tense because of a lack of use. Yes, the night before, I asked myself, "Do I need a brush and floss?"Caving In Do you know how weird your teeth were after you take off your braces? Perhaps your arm leg when the doctor has taken your cast?

That's how my stomach felt heavy the last morning of my three days. It had deflated overnight and felt completely weird to me. In my hand, I couldn't stop touching it. Usually, I can do that stupid trick of poking out my stomach like I'm pregnant, but I can't.

It wasn't injured or anything. It just felt a little closer than usual, in the right way.

HOW TO GET MOTIVATED ON 7 DAYS INTERMITTENT FASTING 16/8

I don't follow the plan, and I don't count the calories. I watch what I'm doing, and I'm restricting processed foods. Yet lately, I haven't always made the best food choices. Since I was in the mid-30s, my body seems to be much less accommodating of snack foods. I needed a rebuild.

You've probably heard about intermittent fasting advantages and how the culinary strategy deals with combat infections or removes the weight-loss plateau. Recent studies have found the health benefits of fasting, and I decided to try this out for seven days to see if any of the buzzes are real, from better sleep to slimmer waistline.

Therefore, I switched to the 16/8 form of intermittent fasting: fast for 14 to 16 hours (most of them sleeping), and then restrict my feeding time to 8 to 10 hours. I've spent my meals every four hours of the day and cut out treats, particularly those in front of my bed. I committed to continue my fasting time between 7 and 8 p.m.

Fasting isn't ideal for everyone, and if you have diabetes or other health conditions, you can talk to your doctor before you do anything like this. But you need the motivation to make a healthy lifestyle adjustment, this kind of intermittent fasting may be just what you're looking for.

Getting Started

First of all, I hired my sister to help me to hold me responsible. She has a lot of willpower than I do.

Next, I got ready. I've noticed that menu planning and food preparation are necessary if you want to adhere to a balanced eating plan. I prepared a meal plan for each day over the weekend, shopped and chopped. Each meal required protein, unsaturated fat, and sugar, with plenty of fruit and vegetables. For starters, lunch could be two slices of sprouted grain bread topped with half an avocado, spinach, and two slices of turkey with an apple on the side. Non-caffeinated beverages are recommended for coffee, tea, or low calories.

Dinners needed to be simple, fast, and child-friendly for most evenings. We had things like chicken stir-fry, rice bowls, salmon and sweet potatoes, or crock-pot chicken and vegetables.

My Results Are In

I felt great for the first few days. Instead, when my body adapted and remembered that it didn't have as much sugar, I became a little sleepy. But towards the end of the second week, I started to feel better and see progress. Find out the benefits: I'm Not Hangry When I usually have a snack on carbs or a piece of fruit, I'm dying of starvation about two hours later. I feel shaky, and I get a bit excited. Despite the four-hour interval of meals during these two weeks, shakiness has never occurred. I was starving for the next day, but I was just hungry enough to want to eat that huge, full meal.

More extreme responses to hunger, such as jitters, irritability (or hanging), and frustration, are caused by a decrease in blood sugar. It often happens to people with diabetes. But even without diabetes, many of us find that a shift in mood comes to us when it's time to eat. It seems like consuming bigger, nutrient-dense meals helped me to keep my blood sugar steady throughout the day, and I didn't experience those more extreme drops.

Learn to Listen to Hunger Cues. Part of my poor food choices is because I'm feeding out of hunger. Understanding that I set a goal, and a meal plan made me wonder if I was starving because I had a granola bar. Listening to my body's hunger, cues only made me eat when I felt I needed it, or when it was impossible to keep my four-hour schedule. I have made better choices, going for food that gives my body more nutrients and regulates blood sugar like almonds, veggies, and hummus instead of empty calories like chips or crackers.

Body improvements While weight loss was not a primary goal, and I gained nearly two pounds and about half an inch away from my hip. Even a minimal weight loss will help your body better regulate insulin and avoid diabetes. With many family members battling diabetes, I'm looking for ways to reduce my risk.

Must Night This has been a shock. Most of the nights, I toss and turn for a long time before I fall asleep. And in the middle of the night, I still wake up. When I stopped eating after dinner, I fell asleep faster and slept longer than I had in years. Less sleep helps me to concentrate better when functioning, and it's the key to preventing chronic illness.

I love sweets, and when I get thirsty, I crave them more. But, as I packed my plate with food such as avocados and bacon, I found that I didn't want candy as much. My sister found many of the same advantages, and she had more stamina and noticed that it helped to rely on healthy foods.

HOW TO GET MOTIVATED ON 30 DAYS INTERMITTENT FASTING 16/8

I completed a 30-day trial with intermittent fasting, testing the version where one fasts for 16 hours and feeds only for 8 hours every day. I'm going to share in this article what the experience was like.

Of the numerous 30-day trials I did, this was one of the simplest, particularly after the first few days of adjustment. I messed up one day for logistical reasons, eating in a 10.5-hour window that day, but otherwise, it was pretty smooth sailing. I got the food window for a few days within 7 hours. The tightest food period I attempted was about 6 hours.

I've had some prior fasting experience, including 17-day fast water in 2016 and 40-day fast water in 2017, so I've gone for long periods without food since. This didn't take a lot of effort in each event, except for the first few days. The same was true with intermittent fasting, even though I had to keep a watchful eye on the food window every day.

Calibrating the Eating Window

I began this experiment by deciding that I would skip breakfast every day, so my first feeding period was 12–8 pm. It was a good place to start, but in reality, it would be relocated later. As noon rolled around, I'd wrap up whatever research I did first, and then I'd have to prepare something to eat. And when I used this time emotionally, I didn't start eating until 12:30 pm or so.

That was all right, but I didn't like the long stretches of the morning with no sleep, so I didn't need to have dinner too late, because I usually go to bed at 10:30 pm. I got used to skipping breakfast, but I felt like I was doing fine with some food in the morning, mainly when I got up early and practiced.

I tried to move the mealtime to 9 am–5 pm earlier. That was all right, too, but planning with Rachelle to have such an early dinner didn't work well. I didn't feel like I was eating the last meal at 4:30 pm. By the time I was trying this more initial window, I'd already got used to waiting longer for food, and I found it hard to adhere to the previous schedule. My first meal was creeping inevitably later anyway.

Finally, I fell into a routine that I liked, even though I changed it a little. I'd only wait until after 10 am for the first breakfast. By the time I take the first bite of food, it was usually about 10:30 am, which allowed me until 6:30 pm to finish the meal. It was an excellent opportunity, and it didn't feel like waiting so long to get up early. If I was hungry in the morning, I could have eaten soon after 10 am. But if I didn't feel like I was starving, or if I was deeply involved in my morning job, I might not be able to eat until 11 am or later.

And, after some training and practicing, instead of worrying about the date, I found it easier to worry about the start time, so I didn't go to the first bite of food sooner than 10 am. Once 10 am rolled along, I could quickly make a game of pushing it back a little — by 15 minutes, 30 minutes, or sometimes an hour or more. The downside of putting it back was that I could have dinner later that day if I wanted to.

The Experience

I can't say that this experiment was too good, but it wasn't too bad either. I've heard a lot of hype about this way of eating, but my experience seems pretty dull compared to some.

Many days I feel like I could use something to eat in the morning, but most of the time, those feelings were quickly dismissed. All I had to do was fill my mind with something other than rice. Being wrapped up in a creative project was a game.

When the first meal finally came around every day, I enjoyed it more than average. It felt like breaking a fast, even though it was only 16 hours without food.

I always became more conscious of what I was eating, particularly for the first meal of every day. When I was eating at 10:30 a.m., I'd worry about whether I needed to call it breakfast and have some steel-cut oats with fresh berries and coconut milk or call it lunch and have air-cooked tofu or tempeh salad.

Since this encounter disrupted my former food schedule, it made me think about when to eat and pay more attention to how hungry I was, instead of just feeding because it was the regular mealtime.

Mentally, I did not notice any meaningful improvement by eating this way— no improvements of mental clarity that I can detect, but no deterioration either. Nonetheless, by not having an early meal, I save time on food preparation and cooking, so I was able to get going on my working day faster than I needed to.

Weight Loss

Over the last 30 days, I lost a little bit of weight, just 1.6 pounds. But that's only been the last ten days. For the first three weeks, I've been close to my starting weight all the time. Even so, if that weight loss pace were to be maintained for a whole year, it would be 19 pounds, which is not bad for a reasonably easy-to-maintain strategy.

Eating in 8 hours didn't seem particularly advantageous if I just consumed the same amount of food I would have eaten before. It was shockingly easy to eat the same amount of food for the first few weeks. But then I slowly found that I was eating less food than I had before. And that's when I began to see the nudging of my weight. In the long run, though, I think that this type of intermittent fasting will make it easier to lose weight because you're likely to eat fewer calories this way. After a while, it started to feel more effortful to try packing the same amount of food in 8 hours.

I think the key here was to indulge in this way of eating and not to regulate it. Initially, I was dwelling on those 8 hours, and I was worried about when I was supposed to eat my meals during that time as if I had to pre-decide when to feed. Then, I just focused on getting past 10 a.m. and letting my hunger decide when to feed, and that's when this process got better, and I started to lose a little weight.

Sometimes I didn't seem as thirsty as I was before. I ate a banana with some peanut butter for dinner one night, so I didn't want more than that. Some days, I found that I was going for more extended periods without feeding. I might feel empty inside, but I wasn't starving on my own.

Final Thoughts

For the first 20 days, this experiment was almost pointless. I couldn't see any results, and I was still calibrating to find the right food window for me. It was only in the last ten days that I began to notice a few changes. Since then, I had lined up with a meal period that fit perfectly (about 10:30 a.m. to 6:30 p.m.), and I was left with a simple rule: wait until after 10 a.m. before I had some food.

Overall, I believe that 30 days was too little time to draw any conclusions as to what the long-term effects of this way of eating might be. The findings were modest relative to other food studies I've done over the years. The transitions from dairy to organic were much stronger and more visible (like losing 7 pounds in the first week when my body finally lost years of milk clogging).

Nevertheless, this encounter made me curious about intermittent fasting, so I'm likely to continue playing with it. Several people suggested that the food window should be shortened even more, say 4 hours or less. And there are several other combinations to use as well.

I like consistency, so I don't plan to be as rigid about intermittent fasting while driving or on a busy schedule, but the ease of not eating before 10 a.m. has worked pretty well, and it seems pretty easy to keep going.

Chapter 13:

How To Choose Foods

Eating during intermittent fasting (IF) may be frustrating. This is because intermittent fasting is not a diet plan, but a method of feeding. Keeping this in mind, DoFasting experts have developed an intermittent fasting food list that will keep you healthy while you're on your weight loss journey.

Intermittent fasting teaches you when to eat, but it doesn't tell you what foods can be included in your diet. Lack of clear dietary guidelines can give a false impression that you can eat whatever you want. Others may find it challenging to choose "appropriate" foods and drinks.

Not only do they hinder your weight-loss plans, but they can also make you more likely to be undernourished or overnourished.

Eat Real Food

It doesn't take a genius to figure this out. Ultimately, man is never going to improve on what God has made.

"Consume a range of nutrient-dense foods and beverages within and across basic food groups while selecting products that restrict the consumption of saturated and trans fats, cholesterol, added sugars, salt, and alcohol." The dilemma is that common sense must contend with a strong trillion-dollar food industry that is bombarding us with advertisements that are designed to make us consume more and more of the worse things.

There is an inverse relationship between nutritional value and income when it comes to food. The more you refine some products, the more you make it profitable. The more it is stored, the less nutritional value it holds. That's why we see stuff like enriched flour. They're trying to put some of the minerals back in that they've been stored. Everything we end up with is a far cry from what God has given us. Packaged and processed food firms waste little effort to push more of their goods into their target market. More than 90% of their merchandise sales are made to less than 10% of their consumers. "In the case of processed food, the desirable 10% consists primarily of people weighing more than 200 pounds and making less than $35,000 per year." No cost is spared to strike any strategic button that matters to the target market. Like a deer captured close to the range of a hunter, the target never has a chance.

Many times, the unhappiness of the cycle threatens the consciences of the $200,000-per-year marketing executives in charge of it. Others also refuse to participate in their focus groups. Instead of addressing their future victims in person, they choose to study documents in the privacy of their workplaces.

One of the major scandals in junk food society is the degree to which its most dedicated advocates ignore the very items they are promoting.

Such food companies are doing something even worse than exploiting low-income, obese, overweight customers for their goods. Once the target enjoys the drug and becomes a consumer, the business chemists guarantee that they will never be content by consuming just a healthy amount of it.

They] have been updated to ensure that "no one can eat just one of them." Such chemical modification induces a great deal of overconsumption, encourages malnutrition, and kills the natural tendency of our taste buds to search for variation in what we consume.

Maybe at this point, you're starting to feel some righteous indignation. We permitted ourselves to be led astray like pigs to the slaughter. I am told again of the words of Jesus, "The robber comes only to steal, and to kill, and to destroy, and I came that they might have life, and have it abundantly" (John 10:10). Such issues aren't meant to shock us. It's our responsibility to educate ourselves so that we learn right from the bad. That takes me back to that point. The only best thing you can do to ensure proper nutrition is to eat predominantly unprocessed whole foods. Real food, non-edible food-like compounds.

If most of your diet consists of real food, you'll get better nutrition and be more comfortable while eating fewer calories. A safe way to make sure you're eating real food is to walk around the store and keep out of the center.

Eating during intermittent fasting is more about being balanced than just dropping your weight quickly. It is, therefore, vitally important to choose nutrient-dense foods such as vegetables, meat, lean proteins, and healthy fats.

The list of intermittent fasting foods will contain:

FOR PROTEIN

The minimum dietary allowance (RDA) for protein is 0.8 grams of protein per kilogram body weight. Your criteria that vary depending on your fitness goals and your level of activity.

Protein helps you lose weight by raising your energy intake, increasing your satiety, and improving your metabolism.

Also, when combined with strength training, improved protein intake helps build muscle. Getting more muscle in your body improves your metabolism because muscle consumes more calories than fat.

A recent study shows that having more muscle in your legs will help reduce the production of stomach fat in healthy men.

The intermittent fasting diet nutrition list includes:

- Poultry and fish
- Eggs
- Seafood
- Dairy products such as milk, yogurt, and cheese
- Seeds and nuts
- Beans and legumes
- Soy
- Whole grains

FOR CARBS

According to the American Dietary Guidelines, 45 to 65 percent of your daily calories will come from carbohydrates (carbs).

Carbs are the primary source of energy for your body. The other two of them are protein and fat. Carbs come in a variety of ways. Sugar, fiber, and starch are the most popular of them.

Carbs often get a bad rap because it causes weight gain. Not all carbs are created equal, however, and they are not necessarily fattening. Whether or not you gain weight depends on the type and quantity of carbohydrates you consume.

Make sure you pick foods that are high in fiber and starch but low in sugar.

A 2015 study suggests that consuming 30 grams of fiber per day can cause weight loss, increase glucose levels, and lower blood pressure.

Getting 30 grams of fiber out of your diet is not an uphill struggle. You will get them by consuming a basic egg sandwich, Moroccan chicory rice, peanut butter pie, and chicken and black peas enchiladas.

The list of intermittent fasting foods for carbs includes:

- Sweet potatoes

- Beetroots

- Quinoa

- Oats

- Brown rice

- Bananas

- Mangoes

- Apples

- Berries

- Kidney beans

- Pears

- Avocado

- Carrots

- Broccoli

- Brussels sprouts

- Almonds

- Chia seeds

- Chickpeas.

FOR FATS

According to the 2015-2020 Dietary Guidelines for Americans, fats are expected to contribute 20% to 35% of your daily calories. Saturated fat should not add more than 10% of calories per day.

Fats can be good, evil, or just in-between depending on the type.

For example, trans fats increase inflammation, reduce "healthy" cholesterol levels, and increase "poor" cholesterol levels. We are used in fried food and baked goods.

Saturated fats can increase the risk of heart disease. Nonetheless, there are varying expert views on this. It's a good idea to eat them in moderation. Red meat, whole milk, coconut oil, and baked goods contain high levels of saturated fat.

Healthy fats are monounsaturated and polyunsaturated fats. Such fats can reduce the risk of heart disease, lower blood pressure, and lower-fat blood levels.

Olive oil, peanut oil, canola oil, safflower oil, sunflower oil, and soya oil are rich sources of these fats.

The list of moderate fasting foods for fats includes:

- Avocados

- Nuts

- Cheese

- Whole eggs

- Dark chocolate

- Fatty fish

- Chia seeds

- Extra virgin olive oil (EVOO)

- Full-fat yogurt.

FOR A HEALTHY GUT

A growing body of evidence shows that your digestive health is the secret to your overall health. The stomach is home to billions of bacteria known as the microbiota.

Such bacteria affect your intestines, your metabolism, and your mental health. These may also have a vital role to play in many psychiatric illnesses.

You can take care of those tiny bugs in your stomach, particularly when you're fasting intermittently.

The list of intermittent fasting foods for healthy intestines includes:

- All vegetables
- Fermented vegetables
- Kefir
- Kimchi
- Kombucha
- Miso
- Sauerkraut
- Tempeh

In addition to keeping your gut healthy, these foods can also help you lose weight by:

- Decreasing the absorption of fat from the gut.
- Increasing the excretion of ingested fat through stools.
- Reducing food intake.

FOR HYDRATION

According to the National Academies of Sciences, Engineering, and Medicine, the daily fluid requirement is:

- About 15.5 cups (3.7 liters) for men.
- About 11.5 cups (2.7 liters) for women.

Fluids provide liquids as well as food and drinks containing water.

Staying hydrated during intermittent fasting is essential to your wellbeing. Dehydration can cause headaches, extreme tiredness, and dizziness. If you're already dealing with these side effects of fasting, dehydration will make them worse or even more severe.

The intermittent fasting food list for hydration include:

- Water

- Sparkling water

- Black coffee or tea

- Watermelon

- Strawberries

- Cantaloupe

- Peaches

- Oranges

- Skim milk

- Lettuce

- Cucumber

- Celery

- Tomatoes

- Plain yogurt.

Ironically, drinking a lot of water can also help with weight loss. A 2016 review study shows that proper hydration will help you lose weight by:

- Decreasing appetite or food intake.

- Increasing fat burning.

Foods To Exclude From The Intermittent Fasting Food List

- Processed foods

- Refined grains

- Trans-fat

- Sugar-sweetened beverages

- Candy bars

- Processed meat

- Alcoholic beverages.

Combining Intermittent Fasting with Specific Diets: Things to Know

Many people believe that mixing IF with other diets, such as keto diets or vegetarian diets, is more effective in weight loss. That said, the jury is still out on whether this is valid or not. Do you want to try the mixture of IF and keto diet? Make sure you include the following in the high-fat low-carb diet with intermittent fasting foods:

FOR FATS (75% OF YOUR DAILY CALORIES)

- Avocados

- Nuts

- Cheese

- Whole eggs

- Dark chocolate

- Fatty fish

- Chia seeds

- Extra virgin olive oil (EVOO)

- Full-fat yogurt

FOR PROTEIN (20% OF YOUR DAILY CALORIES)

- Poultry and fish

- Eggs

- Seafood

- Dairy products such as milk, yogurt, and cheese

- Seeds and nuts

- Beans and legumes

- Soy

- Whole grains

FOR CARBS (5% OF YOUR DAILY CALORIES)

- Sweet potatoes

- Beetroots

- Quinoa

- Oats

- Brown rice

The food list for intermittent fasting vegetarian diet includes:

FOR PROTEIN

- Dairy products such as milk, yogurt, and cheese

- Seeds and nuts

- Beans and legumes

- Soy

- Whole grains

FOR CARBS

- Sweet potatoes

- Beetroots

- Quinoa

- Oats

- Brown rice

- Bananas

- Mangoes

- Apples

- Berries

- Kidney beans

- Pears

- Avocado

- Carrots

- Broccoli

- Brussels sprouts

- Almonds

- Chia seeds

- Chickpeas

FOR FATS

- Avocados

- Nuts

- Cheese

- Dark chocolate

- Chia seeds

- Extra virgin olive oil (EVOO)

- Full-fat yogurt.

What To Drink During Intermittent Fasting

Beverages can be a lifesaver when it comes to fighting hunger pangs and cravings in your fasting hours. Some drinks can help improve the results of your intermittent fasting strategy. Nice, nice!

Here are the drinks you can enjoy in your fasting windows:

Water

You will (and should!) drink water during your fasting periods. Water is always a great choice, all day long. It could be still or dazzling, no matter what you like. You can also add a lemon (or lime) squeeze to your drink if you want lemon water. Consider infusing a pitcher of water with cucumber or orange slices for other exciting taste combinations.

Yet make sure you stay away from any artificially-sweetened water enhancers (such as Crystal Light). The artificial sweetener will interfere with your rhythm!

Coffee

Black coffee is a calorie-free product that does not affect insulin levels. During the fasting hours, you should drink regular coffee (caffeinated) or decaf coffee, don't add any sweetener or sugar. Spices like cinnamon are all that!

Most coffee drinkers enjoy a cup of joe, or even espresso, in fasting periods with no adverse effects. But some people have a pounding pulse or an upset stomach as they drink coffee in fasting hours, so watch your own experience.

Bonus: Black coffee may enhance some of the benefits of intermittent fasting, and it's quite popular with people who also adopt a keto diet. This research has shown that taking caffeine will help with the development of ketone. Coffee has also been shown to improve long-term stable blood sugar levels.

Bone Broth

Bone broth (or vegetable broth) is recommended at any time you decide to fast for 24 hours or more.

Beware of frozen broths or blocks of broth! These have lots of artificial flavors and preservatives that will counteract the effects of your speed. A good homemade soup, or a foundation of confidence, is the way to go.

Tea

Help increase your satiety with tea, of course! It could just be the secret weapon that makes the fasting strategy simpler but also more effective.

All kinds of tea are perfect for a quick drink, like white, black, oolong, and herbal teas. Tea increases the efficacy of intermittent fasting by encouraging digestive health, probiotic balance, and cellular safety.

Green tea, in particular, has been shown to help increase satiety and promote healthy weight management.

Apple Cider Vinegar

Drinking apple cider vinegar has several health advantages, and you can continue drinking it while fasting intermittently, even during fasting periods. And since ACV helps promote healthy blood sugar and digestion, it may also improve the benefits of your intermittent fasting strategy.

If you're not a fan of apple cider vinegar, use it as a salad dressing while you're chewing glass. It's perfect for you at every time of the day.

Are there any drinks that you should stop during intermittent fasting?

There are a few drinks (including "zero-calories") that you may not know are capable of "breaking the fast." That means that if you eat them, you're going to get your body out of the "hot zone."

Chapter 14:

Importance Of Healthy Lifestyle

Living is all about consensus. Okay, if you believe that you can ignore your bad eating habits just because you exercise regularly, think again. A mistake more people make is to believe that if you lose a lot of calories in the gym, you can eat whatever you want. And, if you're "naturally" thin, you don't have to watch what you're doing. Sadly, trading an hour in the gym for a greasy double cheeseburger or depending on a high diet to take the place of healthy eating habits completely misses the point of living a healthy lifestyle the most important thing you can do is to eat well. Evite contaminants in your diet as much as possible and drink plenty of fresh fruit, vegetables, and whole grains; exercise regularly a few days a week; avoid smoking, even second-hand smoke; and avoid adding too much weight (which should come naturally if you eat well and exercise). While it is not necessarily possible to eat all organic food-the EEC suggests 12 organic fruits and vegetables because of their higher levels of pesticide residues.

Our modern lifestyle is very convenient, but it can also be very unhealthful. Most people eat too many processed foods and too few fruit and vegetables; we never exercise, and when we encounter chronic conditions such as diabetes, we rely on prescription drugs to make us feel better-but these medications often have harmful side effects. Instead of acknowledging the value of living a healthy lifestyle for us and future generations, we perpetuate our bad habits-and then taking potent, dangerous drugs to treat our last symptoms.

Of example, not all facets of a healthy lifestyle are in our power. We will be exposed to certain environmental toxins, whether we like them or not. But many of these variables are totally beyond our influence. Whenever we can, we need to be cautious and make the right choices.

That's why it's so important to be sure that you're eating well as a critical factor in keeping a healthy lifestyle.

Eating a healthy diet is far from essential, simply because people are very complex beings. They may have it in the back of our minds that they consume to sustain our bodies, but we make the majority of our food choices based on their pleasure aspect. Eating is such a pleasant experience that we often choose to eat food that tastes very nice, but that doesn't make us feel very well afterward. They also love these things so much that they eat more than our bodies require, which leaves us overweight, sad, and stressed.

You know that a healthy lifestyle, such as eating right, exercising, and eliminating harmful substances, makes sense, but have you ever stopped thinking about why you pursue them? Every activity that supports your physical, behavioral, and emotional health is a healthy habit. Those activities should enhance your general well-being and make you feel good.

Healthy lifestyles are challenging to develop and often require a change of mind. However, if you're willing to make sacrifices to improve your health, the effect can be far-reaching, regardless of age, race, or physical ability. Here is the value of a healthy lifestyle.

Controls weight

Eating right and exercising regularly will help you avoid excess weight gain and maintain healthy body weight. Getting physically active is key to meeting your weight-loss aim. Even if you're not trying to lose weight, regular exercise will enhance your cardiovascular health, strengthen your immune system, and increase your stamina.

Prepare for at least 150 minutes of moderate physical activity each week. When you can't dedicate this amount of time to fitness, search for an easy way to increase movement throughout the day. For starters, try walking instead of driving, take the stairs instead of the elevator, or pacing while you're talking on the phone.

Eating a healthy calorie-driven diet can also help control weight. If you start your day with a healthy breakfast, you stop being too hungry later, which might send you off to get fast food before lunch.

Skipping breakfast will increase blood sugar, which decreases fat storage. Such foods, which are low in calories and rich in nutrients, help to control weight. Reduce the use of sugary drinks, such as sodas and fruit juices, and choose lean meats such as tuna and turkey.

Improves mood

Doing right with your body pays off for your mind as well. The Mayo Clinic states that physical activity increases the development of endorphins. Endorphins are brain chemicals that make you feel better and more comfortable. Eating a healthy diet as well as exercise will lead to a better body. You're going to feel better about your looks, which can improve your confidence and self-esteem. The short-term benefits of exercise include decreased depression and increased cognitive function.

It's not just diet and exercise that leads to a better attitude. Social connections are another healthy habit that leads to better mental health. Either volunteering, joining a club, or taking part in a film, social tasks help to improve morale and mental functioning by keeping the mind active and the amount of serotonin controlled. Don't just remove yourself. Spend time with your family or friends regularly; if not every day. If there is a physical barrier between you and your loved ones, using apps to stay connected. Pick up your phone or start a video chat.

Combats diseases

Healthy habits help prevent such aspects of health, such as heart disease, stroke, and high blood pressure. You will keep your cholesterol and blood pressure within a safe range if you take care of yourself. It keeps your blood flowing steadily, reducing the risk of cardiovascular disease.

Regular physical activity and a proper diet can also avoid or allow you to control a wide range of health issues, including:

Metabolic syndrome

Diabetes

Depression

Certain types of cancer

Arthritis

Make sure that you book a physical exam every year. The doctor will monitor the weight, pulse, and blood pressure, and take a sample of your urine and blood.

Boosts energy

Since overeating unsafe food, we've all felt a lethargic sensation. If you eat a balanced diet, your body gets the fuel it needs to control its energy level. A healthy diet includes the following:

Whole grains

Lean meats

Low-fat dairy products

Fruit

Vegetables.

Regular physical training also increases muscle strength and endurance, giving you more capacity, says Mayo Clinic. Exercise helps bring oxygen and nutrients to your tissues and gets your cardiovascular system to work more efficiently so that you have more time to do your daily work. It also helps to boost efficiency by encouraging better sleep. It allows you to fall asleep quicker and get a deeper sleep.

Insufficient sleep can give rise to a variety of problems. Apart from feeling tired and sluggish, if you don't get enough sleep, you may also feel irritable and moody. Also, poor sleep quality may be responsible for high blood pressure, diabetes, and heart disease and may even shorten your life expectancy. To improve the quality of sleep, adhere to the routine where you wake up and go to bed at the same time every night. Reduce the intake of caffeine, restrict the napping, and build a comfortable sleeping atmosphere. Turn off the lights and the Radio, and keep the room temperature high.

Improves longevity

Once you adopt healthy habits, you increase your chances of a longer life. The American Exercise Council conducted an 8-year survey involving 13,000 men. The study showed that those who exercised just 30 minutes a day significantly reduced their chances of dying prematurely compared to those who practiced occasionally.

Looking forward to more time with your loved ones is reason enough to keep going. Start with quick5-minute walks and gradually increase the time to 30 minutes.

Strive For A Healthy Lifestyle

It's commitment and not always enjoyable, so why worry? At some point in your life, you will face the revelation that your body's health is the determining factor in what kind of lifestyle you will live. Just as a smoker faces a possible future of emphysema and lung cancer, if you lack healthy eating habits, not only do you face a possible future of overweight or obese, you always run the risk of insomnia, heart disease, diabetes, stroke, digestive problems and more. The choices you make every day–from what to eat for breakfast and whether or not to have an extra slice of pie–affect how you feel and how you act, which, as you may be able to guess, changes everything you do. Choose carefully, and eventually, you will realize that feeding your body well turns into a better, safer, more enjoyable life.

When you agree that learning healthy eating habits is worth it to you, it's time to make some adjustments to your eating. Dare yourself to come up with some new healthy eating habits every day and put them to good use, including drinking more water or using mustard instead of mayonnaise on your sandwiches. Rather than trying to cut out all the "bad" things you're currently eating, such as many processed foods, cookies, soda, candy, and other junk foods, it's much more comfortable and safer to start putting more healthy meals, such as fresh fruits and green vegetables, whole grains, lean meats, low-fat dairy products, nuts, and legumes. This way, you're slowly replacing your bad diet with a proper diet, and you're not left with a big, gaping void where your bad food was once. Once you start filling in healthier foods, it's harder for you to let go of some of the more common dangerous foods.

Tips for Beginning a Healthy Lifestyle

1. Prepare the routine of workouts. Prepare your weekly schedule just like you do with college. Consider your safety and yourself a priority. Schedule training sessions daily just as you would have a fitness group. Commit to your exercises.

2. Get a mate of your exercise. Family and mates are a great place to get going. Getting a fitness partner will help motivate you, drive you, and lead you through workouts. Working with someone else helps to keep you accountable. You're more likely to stay on board when someone else is counting on you for an exercise.

3. Find a class that will inspire you. What kind of exercise is going to get you to the gym? The most important thing at the outset and throughout your healthy lifestyle is to engage in activities and events that inspire you to walk around. Would you enjoy aerobic dance classes, body sculpting courses, or a boot camp at the local gym? Determine the thing that you would like to do the most and gravitate to that task. Sessions are a perfect way to get started. Classes provide a coach to help motivate you to keep your exercises healthy to avoid injury.

4. Get active in a group or game. Have you dreamed of getting involved in activities like basketball, pool, baseball, softball, or running a club? Organized sports events and clubs provide an excellent environment for engaging with like-minded people. Sporting organizations and activities are the best way to keep you involved, motivated, and on a training schedule.

5. Set short-term and long-term goals. First and foremost, it's essential to be realistic about your goals. If your goals are to lose weight, boost fitness, compete in athletics, or just become more social, goals can be a great way to keep you on track. Make sure you monitor your success as well. Whether you're checking on your milestones or making a diary or using an app on your phone, keep track of the actions you're doing to achieve your goals

and by what date you'd like to achieve your goals. That person is different, and the expectations of each person should be unique to you and your health and lifestyle.

6. Adopting healthy eating habits. Not only are the workouts important, but healthy eating is also essential. If you want to boost your fitness, lose weight, and become safer, you'll need to fuel your body properly. Make sure you hydrate, eat whole fresh foods and try to remove processed foods from your diet. Prepare your weekly menus, log your diet every day, and note to thank you for all your hard work at the end of each week. Note, it's about lifestyle, not poverty.

A healthy lifestyle is not going to happen overnight. But with a regular exercise schedule, healthy eating, and healthy eating habits, you're one step closer to your target. Sit down and work out a workout schedule and a healthy eating schedule. Getting organized will help you stay on track and make sure you stick to your new healthy routine.

Healthy Lifestyle Make Differences

Okay, as it turned out, a healthy lifestyle makes a big difference. According to this study, people who met requirements for all lifestyles lived substantially, impressively longer lives than those who did not have: 14 years for women and 12 years for men (if they had this lifestyle at the age of 50). People who did not have any of these patterns were much more likely to die early from cancer or cardiovascular disease.

The authors also measured life expectancy from how many of these five healthy habits people have. Just one healthy lifestyle (and it doesn't matter which one) only one extended life expectancy of men and women by two years. Not unexpectedly, the healthier lifestyle people have longer their lives.

Okay, this is massive. However, it supports earlier, similar research— a ton of earlier, related research. A 2017 study using data from the Health and Retirement Study found that people 50 and older, who were of normal weight, had never drunk and had regularly drunk alcohol, lived an average of seven years longer. A 2012 mega-analysis of 15 international studies comprising more than 500,000 people showed that more than half of early deaths were due to unhealthful lifestyle factors such as poor diet, inactivity, obesity, excessive alcohol consumption, and smoking. And the list of research aids continues.

Chapter 15:

Importance Of Regular Weight

When you grow older, if you continue to eat the same kinds and amounts of food but do not become more involved, you are likely to gain weight. That's because your metabolism will slow down with age, and body composition may be different from when you were younger.

The nutrition that the body derives from the nutrients in the meals you consume is known as calories. As a rule of thumb, the more calories you consume, the more healthy you have to keep your weight. Likewise, the reverse is true— the more involved you are, the more calories you use. The bodies may need less food for energy when you mature, but it still needs the same amount of nutrients.

Decreased Breast Cancer Risk

Overweight can increase the chances of breast cancer by 30 to 50 percent, according to the Cancer Prevention Organization.

Improved Heart Health

A record published in the Journal of the American College of Cardiology, which looked at almost 15,000 relatively stable Korean individuals with no documented heart disease, shows that those with the body mass index (BMI) of more than 30 were more likely to show signs of early plate build-up in their arteries than normal-weight people. This has prompted researchers to believe that, although these individuals may have been metabolically stable at the time of the test, their weight is likely to have negative consequences on their health still.

More Motivation

A study of Obesity shows that overweight women's brains respond negatively to the idea of working out— but that people's photos favorably influence women's brains that are at a healthy weight in the middle of a workout session.

Increased Fertility

The ideal weight — in terms of pregnancy — is the BMI between 20 and 24, say, fertility experts. The American Society for Reproductive Medicine currently reports that 12% of cases of infertility are due to weight-related problems (about the same number of people who have infertility are overweight and underweight). Why? Why? Your weight will affect your cycles and ovulation— so if you don't have a regular beating, your fertility can fail.

Better Sleep

According to a 2012 study, weight loss— particularly nasty abdominal fat — may help you record higher-quality fat. Fat, and specifically belly weight, interferes with lung function, making it harder for the lungs to expand because fat is in the way. And since breathing problems can lead to nighttime complications such as sleep apnea, it takes a toll on your eyesight.

Decreased Risk of Diabetes

In those who are overweight, only slight weight loss is linked to delaying — or preventing — diabetes;

More Birthday Candles

It's no secret that people of normal weight are at a higher risk of disease and therefore live longer. But do you know for how long? The risk of death rises by around 30 percent for every 33 pounds of excess weight. The lifetime of an obese person (anyone with a BMI of 40-45) is up to 10 years less than that of a normal-weight person.

How To Keep A Regular Weight

Many factors can influence your weight, including biology, age, gender, diet, family and community, sleep, and even where you live and work. Some of these aspects can make it difficult to lose weight or to keep weight off.

But being busy and eating healthy foods has health benefits for everyone, regardless of age or weight. It is essential to choose nutrient-dense foods and to be active for at least 150 minutes per week. In the thumb rule:

- To maintain your weight the same, you need to consume the same amount of calories as you eat and drink.

- To lose weight, consume more calories than you eat and drink.

- To gain weight, consume fewer calories than you eat and drink.

Maintenance For RegularWeight

Reduce portion size to monitor calorie intake.

Add healthy snacks throughout the day if you want to get more weight.

Physically active as you can be.

Talk to your doctor about your weight, whether you find you weigh too much or too little.

Therefore, being healthy will help you live longer, reduce your chances of developing chronic disease, and help you get more out of your life.

Chapter 16:

14-Day Intermittent Fasting Recipes

BROWNIE CHEESECAKE

Brownie cheesecake is a combination of cheesecake (low in carbohydrate) and brownies that are gluten-free. So it is two delicious desserts in one! The amount of carb in this is less than 0.5g per serving.

Ingredients

Almond flour or coconut flour (that is finely ground)

Butter (soft): grass-fed butter should be used because it contains more healthy fats (omega 3 fatty acids) and has a higher micronutrient level than regular butter. Also to make the butter soft, keep the butter for about 40 minutes at room temperature. This helps to loosen the consistency of the butter and make it soft.

Erythritol (the powdered form): this sweetener is used in keto desserts because it is keto diet friendly as it does not raise the blood sugar level and it is very safe to use.

Cocoa powder: Dutch baking cocoa powder): it is used because just a small amount is needed to achieve a great chocolate taste and flavor and helps to achieve a low carbohydrate recipe.

Vanilla extract (that is free of sugar)

Cream cheese (the full-fat type)

Some chocolate bars (to be grated)

Tools/ Utensils Used

Fridge/ freezer

Parchment paper to line the silicone molds

Mixing bowls

Big spoon

Greater

Silicone molds

Preparation

For The Brownie Layer

Mix the Dutch baking cocoa powder and the vanilla extract in a mixing bowl until it has combined well

Add the soft butter and mix well. (be sure to make the butter mix well in the mixture to form a paste)

Pour the mixture(the brownie layer) halfway into an appropriate silicon mold of the desired size (be sure to fill it halfway so as to allow for the cheese layer to also be poured in it)

The brownie layer can be stored in a fridge pending the time the cheesecake layer would be ready.

For The Cheese Cake Layer

Add the rest of the butter, the almond flour or coconut flour, the rest of the vanilla essence into a mixing bowl and mix till it is very smooth.

When it is very smooth, pour the mixture into the cooled half-filled silicone mold until it is filled up.

Freeze in a freezer for about 2 hours or till it is hard enough.

Remove the already made brownie cheesecake from the silicone mold carefully and serve.

PEANUT BUTTER MOLTEN LAVA CAKE

Nutrition Content In A Serving (One Medium-Sized Cake)

Total Calories: 387 Calories

Calories from fat: 315 Calories

Total Fat: 35.02g

Cholesterol : 215 mg

Protein:10.44g

Carbohydrate:6.41

Fiber: 1.13g

Serving size: 4 servings (4 cakes)

Preparation Time: 25 minutes

Ingredients

2 very big eggs and their yolks

A cup of peanut butter

Chocolate sauce (that is low carb)

Six full tablespoons of almond flour

one full tablespoon of vanilla essence

two tablespoons of coconut oil

seven tablespoons of sweetener (powdered form)

a spoon of butter to grease the baking pan

Tools/ Utensils Needed

oven

baking pan

mixing bowls

a bowl that is microwave safe

spoons

knife

Preparation

Heat the oven to about 370F

Use the butter to grease the baking pan very well so that the cake would remove smoothly without any dent.

Put the peanut butter and coconut oil into a bowl that is microwave safe and stir.

Heat them for a little while to get it melted. When the mixture is already melted, stir it well till it mixes together and is smooth.

Add the powdered sweetener into the melted mixture and whisk it. Also add the almond flour, the vanilla essence, the eggs, and their yolks. Whisk together until the mixture is very smooth.

Fill the baking pan with the batter and bake for about 15 minutes.

Once done, remove the cake from the pan using a knife to loosen the cake from the baking pan.

Place on a serving plate and drizzle it with the chocolate sauce(that is low in carbohydrate)

Follow this process for the four cakes

ITALIAN CREAM CAKE

This cake isn't really Italian as the name implies, never the less it is a great cake that is delicious and also yummy.

Serving size: 4 portions

Preparation Time:

Ingredients

For The Cake

Two cups of almond flour

One cup of coconut flour

One cup of softened butter that is unsalted

4 very big eggs

1 cup of erythritol

A pinch of salt

2 tablespoons of baking powder

One cup of heavy cream

Half tablespoon of cream of tartar

One tablespoon of vanilla extract

One cup of pecans (already chopped)

One cup of already shredded coconut

For The Frosting

Half cup of heavy cream

One cup of soft butter that is unsalted

Two tablespoons of vanilla extract

One cup of cream cheese

Half cup of swerve (powdered)

For The Garnish

Two tablespoons of pecans that are chopped already

Two tablespoons of shredded coconut that are toasted

Tools/ Utensils

Oven

Cake baking pan

Parchment paper liner

Mixing bowl

Preparation

Before starting the preparation, first, heat the oven to about 350F

Use the parchment paper lining to line the inside of the cake baking pan and grease it with a little butter for easy remover

Add the flour, the baking powder, the salt, and the pecans and coconut into a large bowl and stir.

In another bowl, put the sweetener and the butter and cream it until it becomes very fluffy and light.

Remove the yolks from the egg and beat them. Then add to the mixture of sweetener and butter and mix it well.

Then add the heavy cream and the vanilla to the above mixture and mix it very well again.

Add the dry ingredients (the almond flour, the coconut flour, the salt, and the baking powder) into the mixed butter mixture and stir until it is fully combined.

Put the egg whites of the already removed yolk into a bowl and whisk it together with the cream of tartar. Mix it well until it foams.

Then fold this mixture into the already mixed barter. To make the barter light, be sure to fold the egg white mixture lightly.

Pour the batter into the baking pans and bake for about 40 minutes in the already heated oven. By this time, the edges of the cake should be a shade of golden brown and the center of the cake should be firm.

Leave it in the baking pans to cool.

Remove the cake from the pans when they are already cool.

For The Frosting

Put the cream cheese and the butter together in a mixing bowl and start to mix them until the mixture becomes very fluffy and light.

To the mixture, add the sweetener and the vanilla and mix it by beating the mixture.

Next, add the heavy cream to the mixture. To get your desired consistency, add the heavy cream slowly so as to be able to stop when it reaches the desired consistency.

Paste the top of the cake and the side of the cake with the frosting.

On the top layer of the cake, sprinkle the roasted coconut that was shredded and use it to decorate the cake.

GOOEY BUTTER CAKE

Gooey butter cake originated from the United States, from St Louis, Missouri to be precise. The cake is usually dense and flat and also, it usually has a topping of a gooey filling that is sweet and made from butter and cream cheese. The gooey butter cake has three portions: the cake portion, the filling portion, and the sprinkling portion. The cake portion is made with a cake mix that is boxed with a lot of added butter, the addition of lesser eggs, and also no addition of liquids to the cake batter. This is done like that so that it will not rise too much and also so that it will remain buttery and dense. The filling is made by mixing butter, granulated sugar, cream cheese, and egg together by beating it together. Then this mixture is over the top of the cake and then baked till the filling gets gooey. The sprinkling portion is made by sprinkling a desired amount of sugar (or sweetener of choice) on the cake.

Nutrition Content

Total Calories: 268 calories

Calories from fat: 218 calories

Fat: 24. 2 g

Carbohydrates: 4.2 g

Protein: 6.1 g

Fiber: 1.6 g

Portion size: 15 servings

Preparation Time: 60 minutes

Ingredients

For The Cake

Two cups of coconut flour (or almond flour))

One egg

A little salt

Half cup of swerve sweetener

One tablespoon of vanilla extract

Two tablespoons of baking powder

Half cup of butter that is already melted

Two tablespoons of whey protein powder that is not flavored.

For the filling portion

Two cups of already softened cream cheese

One tablespoon of vanilla extract

A cup of powdered swerve sweetener

Two eggs

For The Sprinkling Portion

A cop of powdered swerve sweetener

Tools / Utensils Needed

Oven

Baking pan

Mixing bowls

Stirrer

Preparation

For The Cake Portion

Before starting the preparation process, heat the oven to about 325F

Grease the inside of the baking pan to be used. Grease it with butter to make the cake remove easily.

Put the almond /coconut flour, the baking powder, a little salt, the protein powder and the sweetener in a mixing bowl and mix together until it combines. Also, add the egg, the vanilla extract and the butter and mix well till it combines evenly with the mixture. Pour this mixture into the previously greased baking pan halfway.

For The Filling

Mix the butter and cream cheese together in another mixing bowl and mix well by beating them together. Then add the sweetener until it has fully dissolved and combined with the mixture, then add the eggs and vanilla essence till it is very smooth.

Pour the filling mixture into the half-filled baking pan and bake for about 45 minutes. By this time, the edges of the cake are golden brown in color and the center is still jiggling.

Remove the cake from the baking pan and allow cooling. Then remove and place in a serving plate.

Dust or sprinkle the cake with the powdered swerve and cut the cake into equal bars.

PECAN PIE CHEESECAKE

Nutrition Content

Total Calories: 340 calories

Calories from Fat: 279 calories

Fat: 31.03 g

Protein: 5.89 g

Carbohydrate: 4.97 g

Fiber 1.42 g

Serving size: 10 servings

Preparation time: 50 minutes +3 hours to chill

Ingredients

For The Crust

A cup of almond flour

A little salt

Two tablespoons of swerve sweetener in the powdered form

Two tablespoons of melted butter

For The Topping

Two tablespoons of butter

One tablespoon of whipping cream (heavy)

Half a cup of already powdered swerve sweetener

Two tablespoons of yacon syrup

Toasted pecans (whole) to garnish the cake

One tablespoon of vanilla extract or caramel extract

For The Cheese Cake Filling

Half cup of whipping cream (heavy)

One big egg

Half tablespoon of vanilla extract

Two cups of softened cream cheese

Five tablespoons of powdered swerve sweeteners

Preparation

For The Crust

Add the almond flour, the salt and the swerve sweetener into a big mixing bowl and whisk together.

Add the melted butter and stir well until the mixture becomes clumpy.

Put the mixture into a springform pan and press it to the bottom and up the sides of the baking pan. Keep in the freezer during the time to prepare the pecan pie filling.

Pecan Pie Filling

Melt the butter. This can be done by putting it in a small pot and placing it over low heat. Add the yacon syrup and the sweetener into the melted butter and mix it together until they have combined evenly. Add the vanilla extract or chocolate extract and the heavy whipping cream and stir until they have combined fully.

Then add the egg and start to cook it until this mixture gets thick. After about a minute, stop cooking the mixture from the heat and add the salt and pecan and then stir well.

Spread the mixture over the crust's bottom.

For The Cheese Cake Filling

Put the cream cheese into a bowl and beat it until it becomes smooth. Then add the sweetener, the whipping cream, the vanilla extract, and the egg, beating each ingredient as you add each one.

Pour this mixture on the pecan pie filling and make sure it spreads to the edges.

For The Baking

Use a big piece of foil paper to warp the bottom of the springform baking pan. On top of the springform baking pan, out a piece of towel (paper). Be careful not to let it touch the cheesecake. Also, wrap the foil paper around the top of the pan. The essence of wrapping with foil paper is to prevent excess moisture from entering into the cake batter.

Bake the cake in an oven for few minutes and remove the cake from the baking pan and let it cool down. After this, place the cooled cake in the refrigerator and refrigerate it for over 3 hours.

For The Topping

Place a small pot over low heat; put the butter in it to get it melted. Then put the yacon syrup and the sweetener, whisk them to make the mixture combine well, then add the vanilla or caramel extract, stir, also add the heavy whipping cream and stir again.

Drizzle this mixture (the topping) on the cheesecake and use the toasted pecans to garnish it.

CARAMEL CAKE

This cake is basically a vanilla flavored cake that is almond flour-based.

Nutritional Content

Total Calories: 388 calories

Calories from Fat: 314 calories

Fat: 34. 9 g

Protein:9.5 g

Carbohydrate: 7.6 g

Fiber: 3.4 g

Serving Size: 3 servings

Preparation Time: 1 hour 10 minutes

Ingredients

One cup of almond flour

Three tablespoons of coconut flour

Half a cup of almond milk

Three tablespoons of already softened butter

Two tablespoons of whey protein flour(the unflavored one)

A big egg

A cup of caramel source that does not have sugar

A pinch of salt

Half tablespoon of baking powder

Half tablespoon of the vanilla extract

Preparation

To Make The Cake

First of all, heat the ovens to about 375F. Take a baking pan and grease it to avoid the cake getting stuck in it during removal. Place the parchment paper in the baking pan and also grease the parchment paper.

Mix the flours (the almond flour and the coconut flour) in a mixing bowl and whisk in the baking powder, salt, and whey protein.

In another mixing bowl, whisk the sweetener and the eggs together. Stop when the mixture becomes fluffy and white. Beat the butter into the mixture and also beat the vanilla extract in too.

Add the rest of the ingredients into the barter. Remember to beat the mixture very well upon the addition of an ingredient.

Pour the batter into the cake baking pan and let it spread to the edges of the baking pan. Make sure the top of the batter is smoothened and place the baking pan in the oven.

Bake the cake till the color of the edges are golden in color and also till the top of the cake becomes firm. This should take about 25 minutes.

Remove the cake from the baking pan and put it in a flat plate for it to cool down. Remove the parchment paper longing if it sticks to the cake.

KENTUCKY BUTTER CAKE

This type of cake is moist and also contains a butter cake plus a butter sauce that is very sweet and soaks the cake. The major ingredient in this cake is butter. A very large amount of butter is needed to make this cake. The difference between the normal Kentucky butter cake and the keto version is the type of flour used. In the keto version, almond flour is used as against the wheat flour used in the normal version.

Nutrition content of a serving

Total calories: 301 calories

Calories from fat: 244 calories

Fat: 27.07 g

Carbohydrate: 5.54 g

Protein: 7.34 g

Fiber: 2.4 g

Serving Size: 4 servings

Preparation time: 1 hour 30 minutes

Ingredients

For The Cake

One cup of almond flour

Three tablespoons of coconut flavor

A little water

Half cup of soft butter(make the butter soft by placing at room temperature for some time)

2 eggs

Two tablespoons of protein powder

One tablespoon of vanilla extract

One tablespoon of baking powder

Three tablespoons of whipped cream

A pinch of salt

Four tablespoons of granulated swerve sweetener

For The Butter Glaze

Two tablespoons of butter

Half   tablespoon of water

A quarter cup of granulated swerve sweetener

Half tablespoon of vanilla essence

For The Garnishing

One tablespoon of swerve sweetener

Preparation

For The Cake

Preheat an oven to about 350F, get a cake baking pan, add a little butter to it and grease the pan with the butter, then put two tablespoons of almond flour in the pan and dust it with the flour.

Put the dry ingredients (the almond flour, the baking powder, the salt, the coconut flour, and the protein powder) in a bowl and mix them together.

Get another bowl and beat the Swerve sweetener and the butter together until the mixture turns fluffy and very light. Add the vanilla extract and egg to the mixture and beat it together.

Add the first mixture (the almond flour mixture) to the butter mixture and beat together. Then add the whipping cream and the water to the mixture and beat well until it combines very well.

Pour the batter into the already greased and dusted baking pan. Bake it until it becomes firm and the color changes to a golden brown color. This should take about an hour.

For The Butter Glaze

Place a medium saucepan on medium heat, put the butter and the swerve sweetener in the saucepan and let them melt together. Mix this mixture well to make it combine. Also, add the vanilla extract and the water and whisk them well until the mixture is fully combined.

Create holes in the cake in the baking pan. This can be done with a skewer.

Pour the butter glaze on the cake in the baking pan while it is still warm and let the cake with the butter glaze get cooled down in the pan.

Remove the cake from the baking pan and put it on a serving plate. Be careful to use a knife to make the sides of the cake get loosened so as to make the whole of the cake remove without any dents.

While the cake is on the serving plate, use the powdered swerve sweetener to dust the top and the sides of the cake.

The cake is ready to be served. You can serve with sweetened whipped cream and/or fresh strawberries.

TEXAS CHEESECAKE

It is not restricted to the Americans alone as the name implies. It is consumed all over the world and is a great dessert on the keto diet list.

Nutritional Content

Total Calories: 230 calories

Calories from fat: 183 calories

Fat: 20.3 g

Carbohydrate: 5.9 g

Protein: 5.8 g

Fiber: 3.1 g

Serving Size: 4 servings

Preparation Time: 45 minutes

Ingredients

For The Cake

Half a cup of almond flour

Two tablespoons of coconut flour

One tablespoon of swerve sweetener

Half tablespoon of baking powder

One tablespoon of protein powder that is not flavored

Three tablespoons of salt

A pinch of salt

Two tablespoons of water

Two tablespoons of whipping cream

One egg

Two tablespoons of cocoa powder

For The Frosting

Two tablespoons of pecans that are already chopped

Two tablespoons of butter

A little water (about two tablespoons)

Three tablespoons of cocoa powder

One heaped tablespoon of whipping cream

One teaspoon of vanilla extract

Half a cup of swerve sweetener (in the powdered form)

One teaspoon of xanthan gum

Preparation

For The Cake

First of all heat the oven to about 325F before starting the preparation of the cake.

Get a sheet pan (rimmed, about 10 by 15 inches), grease it with butter.

Mix the coconut flour, the almond flour, baking powder, sweetener, salt, and protein powder by whisking it in a mixing bowl. Make sure there are no lumps in the mixture.

Melt the cocoa powder and powder; add a little water till it is fully melted. Do this by putting the cocoa powder and butter in a small pot and place over low heat. When this melted mixture is boiling, remove it and pour it into the mixing bowl with the whisked dry ingredients.

Add the vanilla extract, the eggs, a little water, and cream. Stir them in until they have fully combined together

Pour the batter in a baking pan and spread it in it.

Place in the preheated oven and bake it for about 20 minutes. By this time, the cake should be firm already.

For The Frosting

Put the cocoa powder, the butter, vanilla extract and a little water in a small saucepan. Place it on medium heat and boil it till it simmers. Stir it to make it smooth. Add the vanilla extract and the sweetener (in powdered form) a little at a time and stir it while adding each portion. If there are any clumps in the mixture, stir and whisk it well to make the clumps dissolve.

Add xanthan gum to the declumped mixture and whisk it very well.

Pour the frost on the cake while still warm and sprinkle pecans on the cake. Let the cake cool for about an hour (so as to make the frosting get set)

Serve

CINNAMON ROLL COFFEE CAKE

This keto cake is filled with cinnamon and glazed with cream cheese that is sugar- free. It is gluten-free and also low in carbohydrates.

Nutritional Content In A Serving

Total calories: 222 calories

Calories from fat: 174 calories

Fat: 19.3 g

Protein: 7.2 g

Carbohydrate: 5.4 g

Serving size: 4 portions (a small-sized cake)

Preparation time: 50 minutes

Ingredients

For The Cake

1 cup of almond flour

A quarter tablespoon of already melted butter

A quarter tablespoon of almond milk

A quarter cup of swerve sweetener

Half tablespoon of vanilla extract

1 egg

A pinch of salt

Two tablespoons of protein powder that is unflavored

A quarter tablespoon of baking powder

For The Cinnamon Filling

One tablespoon of cinnamon in the ground form

One tablespoon of Swerve sweetener in the powdered form

For The Cream Cheese Frosting

A quarter tablespoon of vanilla extract

A quarter tablespoon of swerve sweetener

One tablespoon of cheese cream that is already softened

A quarter tablespoon of heavy whipping cream.

Preparation

Get a small baking pan and grease it with butter

Heat the oven to 325F

Put the ground cinnamon in a small mixing bowl and add the swerve sweetener, then mix it very well. When it has mixed well enough, leave it and start to prepare the cake.

Add all the dry ingredients for the cake in a large bowl. This includes the almond flour, the salt, the protein, the baking powder, and sweetener. Mix them well by whisking them together.

Add the already melted butter, the eggs, almond milk, and vanilla extract and stir vigorously as you add the ingredients for easy and thorough combination.

Put about half of the batter into the greased baking pan and spread it. Then add more than half of the prepared cinnamon filling into the baking pan and add the remaining batter on top of the cinnamon filling. Spread it with a spatula.

Bake until the top of the cake is golden brown in color. This should take about 35 minutes.

Remove the cake into a serving plate and let it get cool.

Add cream, cream cheese, vanilla extract, and the powdered erythritol into a bowl and mix together in a small bowl to make the frosting. Beat the mixture well until it is well combined and smooth.

Pipe the frosting on the cooled cake.

PEANUT BUTTER MUG CAKE

It is important to work through the preparation of the peanut butter mug cake quickly because peanut butter thickens the cake batter the longer it waits.

Nutrition Value Of A Serving (One Mug Cake)

Total calories: 210 calories

Calories from fat: 160 calories

Fat: 17.8 g

Protein: 6.4 g

Fiber : 3 g

Serving size: 5 portions (5 mug cakes)

Preparation time: 5 minutes

Ingredients

A quarter cup of peanut butter

A quarter cup of butter

Half cup of almond flour

3 tablespoons of chocolate chips that are sugar-free

Half a tablespoon of vanilla extract

A quarter cup of swerve sweetener

One tablespoon of baking powder

A little water

Two eggs

Preparation

Put the peanut butter and the butter in a bowl that is microwave safe and place in the microwave to melt it. Make use of the melted mixture is smooth.

Put the almond flour, the sweetener and the baking powder in a bowl and mix together by whisking it. Add the melted peanut butter and butter mixture, the eggs, vanilla extract, and a little water and stir it well till it combines. Also, add the chocolate chips and stir them.

Divide the batter into 5 mugs and bake in the microwave for about a minute each. It should be puff and set by this time.

The cake is ready to be served, serve hot

GINGERBREAD CAKE ROLL

Nutrition Value Of A Serving

Calories: 206 calories

Calories from fat: 163 g

Fat: 18.06 g

Protein: 5.68 g

Carbohydrate: 3.99g

Serving size: 4 servings

Preparation Time: 60 minutes

Ingredients

For The Cake

Half cup of almond flour

One tablespoon of ethical approval

A quarter cup of a powdered sweetener

Half tablespoon of grass fed gelatin

One-eighth tablespoon of cream of tartar

A quarter tablespoon of powdered ginger

A pinch of salt

A little cinnamon powder

A quarter tablespoon of vanilla extract

One eight of powdered cloves

One large egg

For The Vanilla Cream Filling

One cup of softened cream cheese

Half cup of whipping cream

Two tablespoons of powdered sweetener

A quarter tablespoon of vanilla extract

Preparation

For The Cake

Heat the oven to 350F before starting the cake preparation process. Place a parchment paper in a baking pan and line the baking pan with it. Use a little butter to grease the sides of the baking pan and also the parchment paper.

Whisk the almond flour, the cocoa powder, the powdered sweetener, ginger, gelatin, powdered cloves together in a medium mixing bowl.

Get another mixing bowl and mix the granulated sugar together with the egg yolk until the mixture gets thickened and the color turns light yellow.

Also, add the vanilla extract and beat the mixture well.

Beat the egg whites and the cream of tartar and a little salt together in another mixing bowl until the mixture becomes frothy. When it is already frothy, add the remaining sweetener and beat it well.

Fold the beaten egg yolks into the beaten egg whites gently. Then fold this into the almond flour mixture. Be careful not to make it deflated.

Make the batter spread into the already greased baking pan and bake for 12 minutes until it springs back when the top is touched.

Remove it from the oven and let it get cooled a little before removing it. You can remove it by using a knife to make the edges loosen. Cover the cake with another piece of parchment paper and also use a kitchen towel to cover it. Put another baking sheet that is large on top of it and flip the cake over.

Peel the parchment paper gently from the cake and also roll up the kitchen towel gently and let the cake cool down.

For The Vanilla Cream Filling

Beat half of the whipping cream with the cream cheese in a mixing bowl. Beat it till it becomes smooth.

Beat the remaining whipping cream and the sweetener in a big mixing bowl. Then add the vanilla extract and the mixture of the whipping cream and beat very well, but do not overbeat it. Keep about half of the mixture to decorate the cake.

Unroll the cake carefully. Let the cake curl up on the ends and do not lay it down flat completely.

Spread the rest of the filling on the cake and roll it up back gently. Do not roll it up back with the kitchen towel.

Place it on a serving plate. Place the seam side down.

Put the remaining cream mixture on the center of the cake in different shapes. You can use an icing pipe to achieve desired shapes.

Keep In the refrigerator.

KETO PUMPKIN CHEESECAKE

Nutrition Value Of A Serving

Total calories: 246 g

Calories from fat: 211 g

Fat: 23. 4 g

Protein: 5.3 g

Carbohydrates: 3.23 g

Fiber: 1.1 g

Serving size: 4 servings

Preparation Time: 55 minutes + chill time

Ingredients

For The Crust

A quarter cup of almond flour

Half tablespoon of melted butter

One tablespoon of powdered sweetener

A pinch of salt

A quarter tablespoon of powdered ginger

A quarter tablespoon of cinnamon powder

For The Pumpkin Cheese Cake

A cup of softened cheese

One egg

Half a cup of softened cream cheese

Half tablespoon of pumpkin pie spice

Three tablespoons of pumpkin puree

Half tablespoon of vanilla extract

Preparation

For The Crust

Whisk the almond flour, the spices, salt, and the sweetener together in a big mixing bowl. Add the melted butter and stir until the mixture becomes clumpy.

Pour the mixture into a springform baking pan.

For The Filing

Beat the softened cheese and the cream cheese together until it combines well. Add the sweetener and stir well until it becomes smooth.

Add the pumpkin pie spice, pumpkin puree, the vanilla extract and combine it well by beating it well. Add the egg and continue beating it until it combines well.

Use a large foil paper to wrap the bottom of the springform pan. Wrap it tightly. Put a paper towel over the pan. Be careful not to make it touch the cake. Then wrap another foil over the cake top. The reason for wrapping with foil is to prevent excess moisture from entering the cake.

Bake the cake for about 30 minutes; bring it to cool it down.

Refrigerate for about four hours. When it is chilled, use a knife to remove the cake.

If you like, you can add a topping of caramel sauce and whipped cream

CANNOLI SHEET CAKE

Nutrition Value Of A Serving

Total calories: 235 calories

Calories from fat: 180 calories

Fat: 20 g

Protein: 6.8 g

Carbohydrates: 6.2 g

Calcium : 2.9 mg

Serving size: 5 servings

Preparation Time: 40 minutes

Ingredients

For The Sheet Cake

Half cup of almond flour

Half tablespoon of vanilla extract

A quarter cup of sweetener

A little water

Two tablespoons of coconut flour

Three tablespoons of melted butter

Two tablespoons of protein powder

One egg

A pinch of salt

Half tablespoon of baking powder

For The Cannoli Cream Frosting

A quarter cup of milk ricotta

Two tablespoons of chocolate chips (sugar-free)

Two tablespoons of softened cheese cream

A quarter tablespoon of vanilla extract

A quarter cup of powdered sweetener

A quarter cup of heavy whipping cream

Preparation

Heat the oven to about 325F. Grease a small jelly roll pan to avoid the cake sticking to the bottom of the pan.

Whisk the almond flour, coconut flour, sweetener, protein powder, baking powder, and the salt in a big mixing bowl. Add the, already melted butter, eggs, water, and the vanilla extract and stir until they have combined very well.

Pour the batter in the already prepared baking pan and spread it so that there is an even distribution of the batter in the baking pan. Bake the bake for about 22 minutes till the color becomes golden brown and becomes firm while touching.

Remove the baking pan from the oven and let cool completely.

COCONUT FLOUR CHOCOLATE CUPCAKE

Nutritional Value Of A Serving

Total Calories: 268 calories

Calories from fat:

Serving Size: 4 servings (4 cupcakes)

Preparation Time: 35 minutes

Ingredients

Four tablespoons of melted butter

Three tablespoons of cocoa butter

Three tablespoons of almond cream that is unsweetened

Two eggs

A pinch of salt

Three tablespoons of sweetener

One tablespoon of baking powder

One tablespoon of vanilla essence

For The Butter Cream

Half cup of sweetener

One tablespoon of instant coffee

Two tablespoons of softened cream cheese

A little hot water

Half a cup of whipping cream

Preparation

For The Cup Cakes

Heat the oven to 370 F

Use parchment paper to line the inside of the muffin tin

Add the cocoa powder, melted butter, the espresso powder, and melted butter together in a big mixing bowl and whisk them together.

Add the vanilla essence and eggs to the mixture then add the baking powder, coconut flour, a pinch of salt and the sweetener, and then beat well to combine it together.

CONCLUSION

Intermittent fasting is a lifestyle that is not only easy and healthy but also enjoys a meal. Although it opposes many of today's views and ideas, there is the evidence behind it. With all these new ideas and diets, you'd think the world would be getting more fit instead of fat at an all-time high. Through research and science, it proves IF works, and if the Romans, the height of fitness, used it to stay fit, why shouldn't we?

Intermittent fasting was successful for short-term weight loss in healthy, overweight, and obese people. Randomized controlled trials with a long-term follow-up duration are needed to ensure commitment to the diet and long-term retention of weight loss without regaining lost weight. Future studies should also include specific population subgroups, such as people with cardiovascular risk factors and type 2 diabetes mellitus, as these patients are more likely to benefit from weight loss that may influence the disease process. In summary, obesity and overweight are an international health issue, and measures such as ADF are needed to help people achieve weight loss.

Now you know what IF is and how it can help you lose weight quickly, comfortably, and seamlessly.

It also involves cycles of starvation, which places the body in a state of fat burning. During the fasting time (usually 16 hours), there are improvements in the body that facilitate increased longevity, cellular regeneration, reduced inflammation, and changes in hormonal body weight regulation. Although it is not suitable for those who are insulin-dependent who require regular meals, intermittent fasting can be reasonably easy to adapt and can be a proper diet for many individuals.

Although this is a "diet," it does not necessarily mean that anyone who practices an intermittent fasting diet is using it to lose weight. Although, indeed, this diet may allow some patients to break through weight-loss plateaus, it also provides a variety of other health benefits and may be helpful for some health conditions.

Made in the USA
Monee, IL
25 May 2023